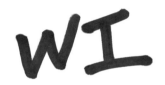

# HOW TO SUCCEED IN
# **BREASTFEEDING**
## WITHOUT REALLY TRYING,
### OR TEN STEPS TO LAUGH YOUR WAY THROUGH

*Published by*

World Scientific Publishing Co. Pte. Ltd.

5 Toh Tuck Link, Singapore 596224

*USA office:* 27 Warren Street, Suite 401-402, Hackensack, NJ 07601

*UK office:* 57 Shelton Street, Covent Garden, London WC2H 9HE

**British Library Cataloguing-in-Publication Data**
A catalogue record for this book is available from the British Library.

Illustrations and cover by Marianna SIMINA
Layout by See More Designs LLC

**HOW TO SUCCEED IN BREASTFEEDING WITHOUT REALLY TRYING**
**or Ten Steps to Laugh Your Way Through**

ISBN-13 978-981-281-915-4
ISBN-10 981-281-915-0

Desk Editor: Tjan Kwang Wei

*Printed in Singapore by Mainland Press Pte Ltd*

NATASHA SHUR, M.D. and PAULINA SHUR, Ph.D.

# HOW TO SUCCEED IN
# BREASTFEEDING
## WITHOUT REALLY TRYING, OR

## TEN
## STEPS
## TO LAUGH
## YOUR WAY
## THROUGH

Illustrations by
Marianna Simina

World Scientific Publishing Co. Pte. Ltd.

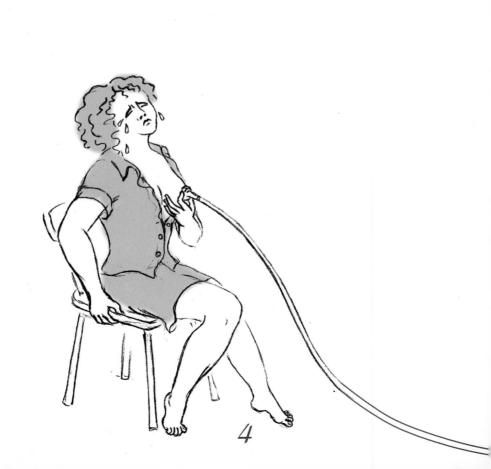

4

# Dedication

*(from Paulina Shur)*

$\mathcal{W}$hen my oldest daughter was born, I developed mastitis. At that time in Russia, where we lived, breast pumps did not exist. The pain in my breasts was so excruciating, I couldn't even think about nursing my baby, but formula was not available. It was a calamity. My husband surveyed the situation. Then, he brought a bicycle pump and made a special connector that stuck to my breast on the one side and to the hose on the other. He went to the opposite side of the room (since the hose was long, and the pump huge and heavy), and started to pump as if my breast were a bicycle's wheel — only the milk was going out, not the air in. I screamed from pain, but in a few minutes most of the milk was gone from my breast, and I was able to nurse my daughter with the remains of the milk in that breast. The same procedure was repeated for the other breast, and this continued every two hours for the next three days. In three days, the mastitis was gone.

When my youngest daughter was born (a co-author of this book), we left Russia. While in transit, we couldn't afford to buy a crib, nor could we put the baby on our bed, for fear of her falling on the floor during the night. My husband surveyed the situation. Then he took one of our huge suitcases, dumped out all of the clothes, put a soft blanket on the bottom, tied both sides of the suitcase to heavy furniture pieces (so that the suitcase wouldn't close while we were asleep), and voila! - a safe and cozy bed was ready for our baby.

To the best husband and father in the world —
Michael Shur

## Thank you:

*To Dr. Nelli Fisher and Dr. Anne Marie Roe who delivered my baby.*

*To my mentor Dr. Marion who has always helped me both personally and professionally and is an inspiration as a pediatrician, geneticist, and person; and my other mentor Dr. Susan Gross for her ideas and brilliance.*

*To Dr. Julie Aliaga, Dr. Kelechi Iheagwara, Dr. Megan Huchko, Dr. Susan Klugman, and Kelly Moffat Saeed for friendship and continued support.*

*To my daughter Anna, the inspiration for this book.*

*Natasha Shur*


## Thank you:

*To my mother, who breastfed me, when I was a baby, and to my husband, who fed me, when I illustrated this book.*

*Special thanks to my Professors: Deanna Leamon (University of South Carolina, SC), Kristina Palana and Thomas Uhlein (William Paterson University, NJ).*

*Marianna Simina*

# THE TEN STEPS

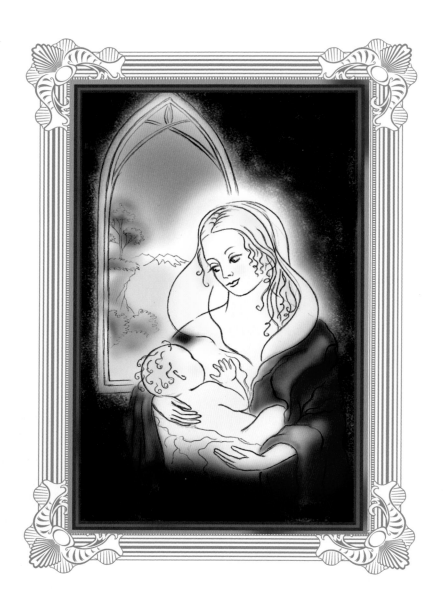

$\mathcal{B}$reastfeeding . . . Doesn't it conjure images of Renaissance women, gently holding their infants, surrounded by the serenity of a landscape – the symbol of eternal harmony between mother and child? Doesn't it remind you of women sitting in cafes or parks, perfectly at ease, chatting with each other, their babies happily feeding?

And yet, when YOU offer your baby your breast for the first time, you scream. You scream from pain and awe. You discover that breastfeeding does not come effortlessly (nor does childbirth). You realize that you are on your own. Neither at the obstetrician's office nor in Lamaze class were you adequately taught the technique of breastfeeding, provided with current information on its advantages, and prepared for its trials and tribulations.

Where is this beautiful woman in the painting, dressed in a rich gown, pensively looking at the distance, while her infant breastfeeds? Your real-life version appears like a battle between you, your breasts, and your child. You weren't prepared for screaming with every feed; crying from ferocious pain (do newborns have teeth?); seeing the milk leaking out of you and staining your shirts; and feeling utmost exhaustion. As one of the obstetricians put it: "It hurt so much, I thought my baby's first word

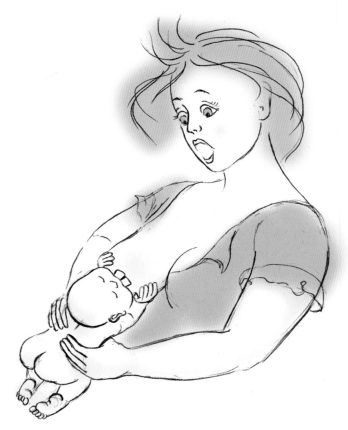

would be F---!" Not surprisingly, only seven out of ten women on average in the United States breastfeed in any capacity, and even fewer by three months of age.[1]

So while Mary's little lamb, or the three little pigs that weren't afraid of the big bad wolf, or mischievous Peter rabbit all suckled their mothers' milk, our baby boys and girls try Enfamil or Similac, Prosobee or Nutramegen,

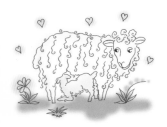
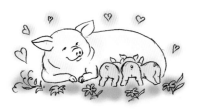
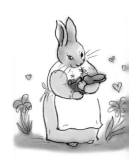

and their mothers still hassle over the formidable task of finding the perfect formula.

But if you come to the hospital mentally and physically prepared, equipped with the right TOOLS for breastfeeding, knowing what to expect, what to demand, and how to fight the sabotages of the hospital system, then not only would you ease breastfeeding in the first few weeks, but soon after you would find yourself sitting on a park bench, the pain subsided, and the baby happily nursing. Breastfeeding would become a beautiful and satisfying experience. Those art images of motherhood are real, after all. It just takes some time and maybe a little help to get there.

This book offers help to women who want to breastfeed (as well as to those who are undecided) and tries to add a little humor to the postpartum period – the most joyful and yet tearful time in a woman's life.

In ten simple steps, this book explains the advantages of breastfeeding; guides you through its problems and obstacles; shows you how to lose weight while sitting on the couch; and saves you enough money to buy a designer dress, go out to dinner at a five-star restaurant, and catch a Broadway show – once you make it out of the house, of course!

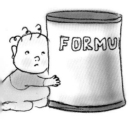

*The* world is so full of a number of things,
I'm sure we should all be as happy as kings.

Robert Luis Stevenson, *Happy Thought*

step one

# CHOOSE NURSING OVER NURSERIES

## *(while pregnant, think breastfeeding)!*

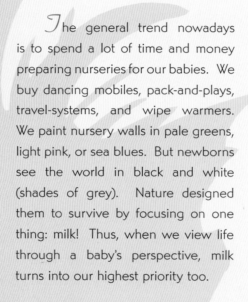

The general trend nowadays is to spend a lot of time and money preparing nurseries for our babies. We buy dancing mobiles, pack-and-plays, travel-systems, and wipe warmers. We paint nursery walls in pale greens, light pink, or sea blues. But newborns see the world in black and white (shades of grey). Nature designed them to survive by focusing on one thing: milk! Thus, when we view life through a baby's perspective, milk turns into our highest priority too.

Just as we take care to choose the right car-seat, crib, and stroller, we should consider the food we offer our baby with the same or even greater care.

12

# To Breastfeed or Not To Breastfeed?

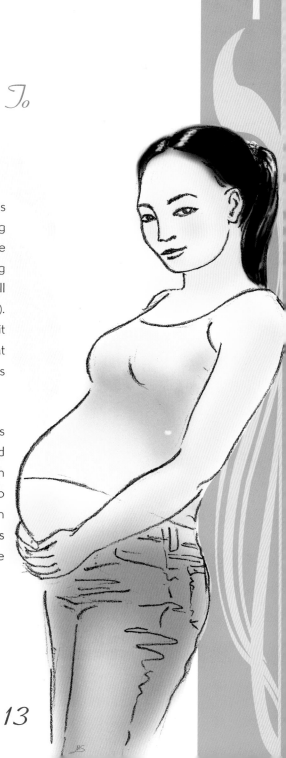

The best time to make this very important decision is during the pregnancy (while you deprive yourself of wine, experience morning sickness and leg cramps, but still manage to make it to the movies). Women who think that they can wait until after delivery and then see what happens with breastfeeding are less likely to succeed.

Breastfeeding certainly offers advantages to you, your baby, and even the baby's father (although the poor man will be relegated to the status of a second class citizen in your heart after the baby is born). It is worth considering the most compelling.

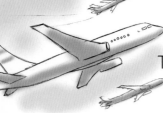

## THE TOP TEN REASONS FOR A MOTHER TO BREASTFEED:

1. Breastfeeding is trendy lately (it was even in Vogue with model Angela Lindvall nursing her toddler son). Stock up on some cute button down shirts for the occasion!

2. Breastfeeding burns up to 500 calories per day (equals at least a guilt-free fudge Sundae).

3. Breastfeeding is over a thousand dollars cheaper than formula feeding: a good breast pump costs between $200-$300 versus a year of formula at over $1,500. Fly away to an all-inclusive resort on the money you save!

4. Mothers who breastfeed have a lower risk of developing breast, uterine, and endometrial cancers.

5. Mothers who breastfeed won't get their period any time soon (although it is a myth that they can't get pregnant; the progestin-only pill, condoms, or an IUD are birth-control options). As a result, they are less likely to get anemia, and they can forget about cramps. Just think, nine or more period-free months!

6. The mother's uterus shrinks faster (breastfeeding outdoes sit-ups).

7. Due to the stimulus of uterine contractions, mothers who breastfeed have a decreased risk of severe postpartum hemorrhage. You recover from delivery faster!

8. Breastfeeding mothers don't have to worry about selecting the best brand of formula for the baby; instead, they can use their limited shopping time buying name-brands (i.e. clothing) for themselves.

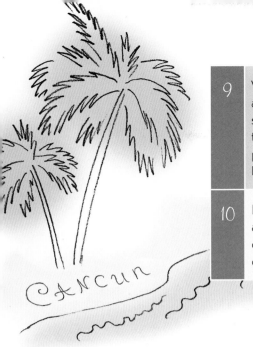

| 9 | Women's breasts start developing and preparing for breastfeeding six weeks after conception! When the baby is born, colostrum (which precedes milk) is already there, begging to be used. |
| 10 | Breastfeeding eventually feels warm and cozy, and offers moments of peace and contentment in an otherwise hectic life. |

My Mama says that I'm her world,
A great big world, you see.
Now don't you think that's funny
When I'm really only me?

She says it's bounded on the North
By a curl (I hate them too),
And that it's bounded on the South
By a very muddy shoe.

And on the East and West it goes
As far as I can reach.
Now isn't that a funny thing
For any one to teach?

My Mama says that I'm her world
By every Mama's Rule.
Of course, I'll learn it differently
When I start in to school.

Anna Bird Stewart, *Geography*

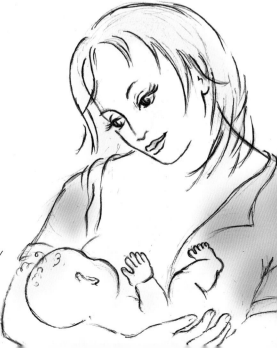

15

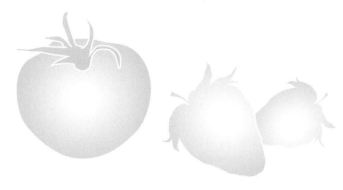

# THE TOP TEN REASONS FOR A BABY TO BE BREASTFED:

**1** Breastfed babies have fewer illnesses, because milk transfers antibodies (IgA) against disease and contains macrophages, which are like scavengers for bacteria, viruses, and fungi. Colostrum, the protein-rich mixture that precedes mature milk, is considered liquid gold by breastfeeding gurus: it is packed with antibodies.

**2** Breastfed babies have a decreased risk of developing food and other allergies. Bring on the strawberries and tomatoes (but just talk to your pediatrician first).

**3** Breastfed babies are far less likely to get hospitalized with pneumonia in infancy.[2]

**4** Breast milk contains endorphins, which work as natural pain-relievers (it is great to breastfeed after the baby gets those two, four, and six month shots!).

**5** Breastfeeding facilitates tooth and jaw development with less dental abnormalities. Isn't it amazing that you can influence your baby's oral-motor structure?!

**6** Breastfeeding works like a pacifier, calming and soothing the baby, and helping fight some stomach aches. You never knew that you would be a live pacifier, did you?

| 7 | Breast milk has the perfect combination of fat, carbohydrates, and proteins for the baby, always has a nice, warm temperature, and tastes better than formula (try a taste test!). |
|---|---|
| 8 | Breast milk is the ultimate organic food. |
| 9 | Breast milk protects the baby against diarrhea. It is the safest food for a little world traveler. |
| 10 | Breastfed baby girls have a slightly decreased risk of developing breast cancer when they are older (the lifelong benefits are awe-inspiring).[3] |

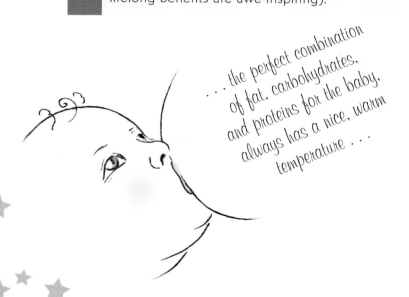

... the perfect combination of fat, carbohydrates, and proteins for the baby, always has a nice, warm temperature ...

My baby has a mottled fist,
My baby has a neck in creases;
My baby kisses and is kissed,
For he's the very thing for kisses.

Christina Rossetti, *My Baby Has a Mottled Fist*

17

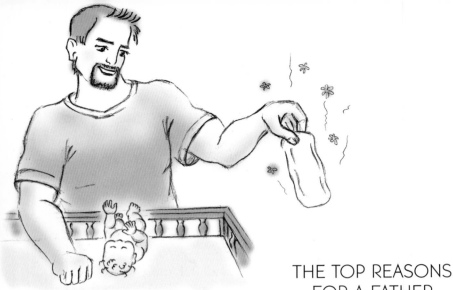

## THE TOP REASONS
## FOR A FATHER
## TO HAVE A BREASTFED BABY:

| | |
|---|---|
| 1 | Breastfed diapers smell a lot better, especially before introducing solids. |
| 2 | The truth is that fathers end up getting more sleep. While they may be on diaper duty, they don't have to run to the kitchen to warm a bottle and feed the baby. |
| 3 | The father will spend on average less time missing work for doctor's visits. |
| 4 | The father has less garbage to take out (formula bottles add up). |
| 5 | Let's face it: the baby might think of the mother as the food-supply; that leaves the father in the happy role of the playmate! |

"*B*y producing milk, my honey,
You are saving time and money.
No to baby histrionics!
Yes to cars and electronics!"

One Father's "*Thank You*"

# The Breast Basics:
## A Little Biology Never Hurts

Did you know that women's breasts begin developing six weeks after conception, two weeks after the heart forms? They start with a "milk ridge," which forms as paired glands running side by side in parallel rows along the fetus' body from above the armpit to the groin. By nine weeks, most of the milk ridge disappears except for two main elevations, which will become the breasts.

When our breasts grow, it is the first sign of puberty. Our bodies change from girlish to womanly. The areolae surrounding the nipple darken and our breasts take on their shapes – round, cone-like, or oval. Breasts become part of our identity and femininity. In many cultures, and for many artists, from Rubens to Picasso, their voluptuousness heralds beauty, womanhood, and sensuality.

For most of our lives, the breasts are hardly considered functional. But when we get pregnant, everything changes. At around seven months gestation, a hormone called prolactin (produced by the pituitary gland) increases and then surges. At that point, milk production (in the early form of colostrum) begins, though we often remain unaware of our newly developed function. The female hormones, estrogen and progesterone, high in pregnancy, keep the growing milk supply in check. After the baby is born, estrogen and progesterone fall, while prolactin reigns – time to make milk!

19

Our breasts do so in an elaborate process. Within the fat of breasts, there are around 15-20 lobes, which contain milk-producing glands called **lobules** (little lobes). The little lobes contain clusters of **acini**, which means grape in Latin. It seems that the Romans thought of breasts as vineyards. Maybe that explains why many Renaissance paintings depict bosomed maidens holding grapes in their hands. While grapes make Champagne, the acini make breast milk. They are connected to stems and larger vines that deposit the milk into **ampullaes** — jugs in Latin — that can pour milk out into the nipple.[4]

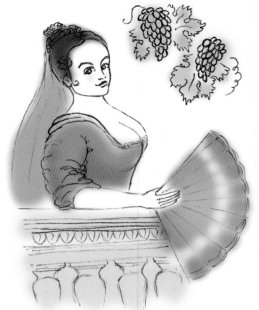

When the baby suckles, the breast becomes erect. People never talk about erections in women, but they happen. They happen as a result of a highly coordinated process known as "the milk-reflex." In other words, the breasts and the brain are connected. The breasts are mostly composed of fat, glands, and an intricate network of nerves. The nerves in the breasts send messages to the hypothalamus — a structure in the brain located in the cerebral cortex (the thinking part of the brain). The hypothalamus regulates body

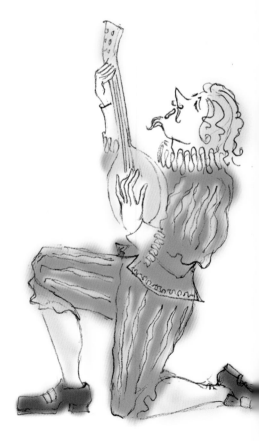

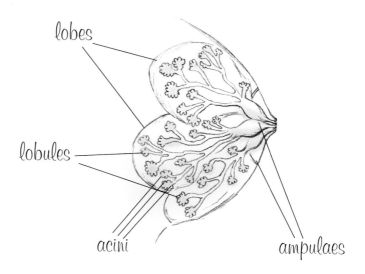

lobes

lobules

acini

ampulaes

functions like sleeping, body temperature, and in the case of breasts, milk production. Then the pituitary gland – another structure in the brain – responds to signals from the hypothalamus by releasing two hormones: prolactin, that causes milk production, and oxytocin, that causes milk release. The oxytocin stimulates smooth muscle cells (myoepithelial cells) around the breast to contract. The milk is "let-down."

It is awe-inspiring to consider the exquisite coordination and interdependence between the brain and the breasts, and a mother and her newborn. Our emotions and thoughts also play a role. Later, oxytocin may be released during lovemaking, or when we hear our babies cry, or even when we think about them. That explains why the woman in the grocery aisle suddenly leaks milk (and when we become her, all we can do is laugh).

# What's in a Rose (or in a Breast)

$W$e spend most of our lives *consuming* food; it is bizarre to consider how we suddenly start *producing* food. The process is called *lactogenesis* (meaning, birth of milk). To understand it, we must have a basic knowledge of genetics.

In each of the cells in our body, we inherit forty-six chromosomes (twenty-three from the mother and twenty-three from the father), which provide a map of our hereditary characteristics. On the chromosomes, there are around twenty thousand genes, which encode the formation of specific functions and proteins in our body. The puffer fish has almost as many genes as we do, but clearly, the genes in every species code for a slightly different product. We now know that genes can be turned on and off in a dynamic process that allows for complex biological responses throughout life. Pregnancy turns the certain genes on, which in turn promote synthesis of $\alpha$-lactalbumin, the predominant sugar in breast milk.

Under a microscope, cells in our breasts before pregnancy appear mainly filled with large fat droplets, and at this point they lack machinery to secrete milk. During pregnancy and immediately after delivery, a combination of maternal hormones stimulates the cells to mature. Breast cells gain an advanced protein-making structure, called the endoplasmic reticulum (ER), and a distribution and shipping department, called the Golgi apparatus (GA). The ER and GA are found in the majority of cells in our body, but they work specifically depending on the needed function: in the case of breast milk production, proteins and lipids that are built in the ER bud off into tiny bubble-like vesicles and float through the cell until they reach the GA, where they are further adapted for the infant. These GA secretions are combined with other nutrients that have floated in through the blood stream. After some additional and highly complex processing steps, breast milk is ready.

It is postulated that maternal hormones promote the dilation of vessels, which leads to increased blood flow towards our breasts. Since our heart pumps blood to the body, we can think of breast milk as coming straight from the heart, both literally and figuratively speaking. Less romantically, we can think of it as coming from our stomachs. The exact supply of nutrients changes slightly depending on what we eat. This is the reason why breast milk might taste differently after a meal of Pasta and Pesto versus a desert of chocolate cake. While milk is a complex fluid with many hundreds of minor components (and immunoglobulins, which protect against disease), the major nutrients include fat, proteins, carbohydrates, ions, and water. It is a *species* specific combination (if not *person* specific). For example, milk in seals and whales has little carbohydrate but a higher concentration of ions. In contrast, milk of primates is low in ions but high in carbohydrates. The exact combination of water, specific proteins (the most common proteins are casein and whey), and lactose differ in humans, cows, blue whales, and every other mammal (see table on the next page).[5]

|  | Water % | Fat % | **Casein %** | Whey % | Lactose % |
|---|---|---|---|---|---|
| HUMAN | 87.1 | 4.5 | **0.4** | 0.5 | 7.1 |
| COW | 87.3 | 3.9 | **2.6** | 0.6 | 4.6 |
| BLUE WHALE | 45.5 | 39.4 | **7.2** | 3.7 | 1.4 |

The above numbers do not add up to a hundred percent, because there are some additional "secret ingredients." The biggest difference between human and cow's milk is that the latter has much more casein protein, which can upset the infant's belly. Thus, formula manufacturers have to modify cow's milk and try to get the casein out, one formidable task among many. That factory process is never perfect. It cannot compete with the intricate manufacturing capabilities of our own cells.

# Formula Companies Compete with Breast Milk in a Different Way

Formula companies bring pens, bags, and lunch to medical staff, and carts of free formula to the pediatric offices and wards. They also make deals with maternity stores to get addresses of pregnant women, and then they send them free formula. Their goal is to make formula a ubiquitous presence in hospitals and homes.

Many women are not aware of the big business side. The price of formula is staggering, although it

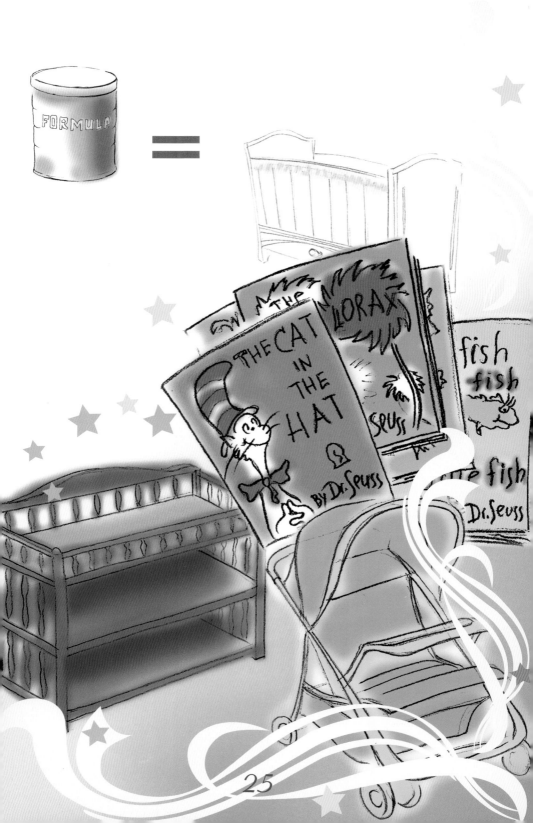

FORMULA =

THE CAT IN THE HAT
By Dr. Seuss

THE LORAX
Seuss

fish fish fish
Dr. Seuss

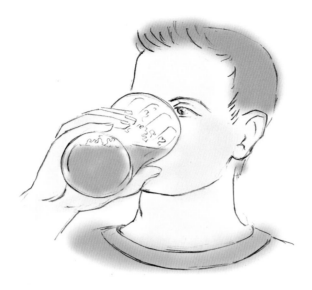

varies depending on whether it is bought in cheaper powdered or more expensive pre-mixed forms and whether it is cow-milk derived, soy, or made from free proteins (up the echelon of formula). The cost for the year (not including bottles or other hidden expenses) for an exclusively formula-fed baby is likely between $1500 - $2500, enough to buy all the baby necessities together: a stroller, car seat, crib, changing table, and plenty of Dr. Seuss books! So a nursing mother could afford her entire nursery! Or she could afford a day in a spa and other luxury items – all well deserved.

One father pointed out that he would rather compare the price of formula to other beverages: the average amount spent on formula could buy five 12-oz glasses of Guinness per day for one year (based on one 50 L keg for $140, for a total of $1800). Ounce per ounce formula is more expensive than premium imported Irish beer.

Like beer-brewers, formula-makers invest a lot of money into making their bottles look attractive (showing cute babies instead of women and sports cars). To further enhance their influence, they use the same strategy as tobacco companies.

It is a well-known fact that tobacco ads appeal to minors. Research has shown that if people begin to smoke under the age of 18, they will become addicted. Formula companies hook people in a similar manner. Research has shown that if women do not start out breastfeeding exclusively, they are unlikely to continue. Thus, formula companies strategize for the cessation of breastfeeding. Women, when exhausted during the postpartum period, may not realize that by accepting something "free" now, they are making a decision for which they will pay (literally and figuratively speaking) later.

There is yet another tactic that formula companies use successfully: the snake-oil salesman tactic. In 2002, a certain premier formula company started marketing advanced brands, supplemented with the two fatty acids – DHA (docosahexaenoic acid) and ARA (arachidonic acid), which are found in small amounts in breast milk. The company claimed that the supplements promote brain and eye development (after reports on breastfed babies suggested that these substances have positive effects)! The formula companies added DHA and ARA to their "premium" brands and made them more expensive. The clever idea is to market towards people's fears that, lest they buy the higher-level formula, their children might not maximize their potentials. The reality is that breastfed and formula-fed babies, even without supplements, may have similar IQ in the long run, and it is a strike against humanity to implicate that extra drops of DHA and ARA create some sort of bell curve for standardized baby intelligence. There are children who get adopted from orphanages where they survived mainly on mush, but after they are placed in loving homes, they flourish. Clearly, many different factors play a role in a child's development, aside from what she eats. If people want to ensure extra IQ points, they are just as likely to succeed by reading *The Little Prince* a few times.

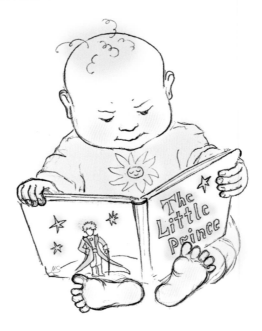

However, research has certainly shown that breastfed babies get sick less often. Most commonly, they get fewer ear infections.

# From Breasts to Ears: Connect the Dots for Your Tots

When I was a pediatric resident working overnight in the emergency room, I saw many sick babies. The parents who brought them had been up for two nights in a row, exhausted and miserable. The babies were feverish and tearful; they had colds, coughs, and they vomited. I would examine them as they coughed in my face (and I have certainly suffered my share of colds afterwards). Their lungs were clear. Their hearts were regular. Their bellies were soft. And then, I would look into their ears, in hopes of seeing the tympanic membranes. On worse days, I would have to dig out wax in the canal, a painful and miserable ordeal, or pour in Colace (a stool softener) drops so the wax would drip out. Normally, the tympanic membranes look like pearls, but now they appeared bright red, and bulging. Tylenol and pink bubble-gum colored antibiotics do wonders for ear infections (although they stain everybody's clothes), and after a few days the babies would feel better. However, it would typically take between four to six weeks for the tympanic membranes to look like normal pearls again (they often appeared like crinkled saran wrap in between). Some of the babies with recurrent ear infections had chronic fluid in their ears, which could potentially cause hearing loss and speech acquisition problems. The management is to place ear tubes, which resemble little white donuts, via a minor surgical procedure which helps the fluid drain. Whatever the result, I knew that if I could possibly prevent an ear infection, I would try it with all my might.

29

Of course, breastfed infants occasionally get ear infections too, and some formula-fed babies never sneeze in their lives, but why take any chances? Any discomfort you experience in the beginning of breastfeeding would work towards possibly preventing misery later. Any sleepless nights at the beginning might minimize crying, irritable nights in the future, for both you and your baby.

There are other cases when breastfeeding may be of paramount importance. This is particularly true for premature infants. Those who receive breast milk have a decreased risk of necrotizing enterocolitis (a life-threatening intestinal complication) and a decreased incidence of sepsis (bacteria in the blood). The breast milk benefits have been so dramatic that some Neonatal Intensive Care Units have begun buying pasteurized donor milk ($3.00/ounce) for infants whose mothers cannot provide pumped milk. It has been calculated that every dollar spent for pasteurized human milk results in a relative saving of approximately eleven dollars in healthcare costs.[6] Clearly, breast milk is valuable for our

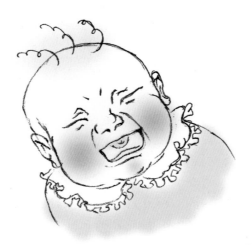

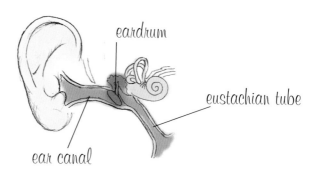

own babies and society in general. For those mothers who have healthy newborns and an oversupply of breast milk, it is rewarding to know that their donations are potentially life-saving.

When you are pregnant, your baby is always with you. After you give birth, and the umbilical cord is cut, there may be moments when you forget that the baby is no longer inside you. You wake up in the middle of the night frantic, your hand on your belly, wondering why the baby is no longer moving. Then you realize that the baby is out, peacefully sleeping next to you. When you breastfeed, you bring back physical attachment and co-dependence between you and your baby. Giving yourself to this tiny little creature is fulfilling. It makes you happy.

**IN SUMMARY:**

There are emotional, medical, biological, and economical advantages to breastfeeding. There are practical ways to make it easier.

# TOP TEN WAYS TO PREPARE TO BREASTFEED DURING PREGNANCY:

1. Ask about the availability of breast pumps in the hospital where you will deliver: some places have pumps in every room - that is definitely a plus! You may still consider bringing your own pump, especially if you need help learning how to use it.

2. Consider buying the best breast pump possible. If you plan a baby shower, consider putting the breast pump on your registry list. Or call your insurance company regarding possible reimbursement (it pays to read the small print).

3. Ask if you can room-in with your baby in the hospital. If you are separated from the baby, put a sign on the bassinet that says, "BREASTFEEDING ONLY – NO FORMULA!" That way, if there is a critical reason to give formula, hospital staff will remember to discuss the plan with you first.

4. Consider taking a breastfeeding class or setting up a personal session with a lactation consultant. This is even more important than learning how to breathe in Lamaze: there is an epidural to help with the pain of labor but little help for the initial pain of breastfeeding.

5. Buy a tube of lanolin (to use around those "sore" nipples) and a bottle of acetaminophen.

6. Find out the number to your local La Leche league (they are unbelievably kind and helpful); put it on the refrigerator and take it to the hospital.

**7** Make a list of your best friends and co-workers who successfully breastfed. Put their numbers on your refrigerator and take them to the hospital.

**8** Buy a few maternity bras. Remember that while you use your pre-pregnancy size to determine maternity clothes, you can't apply the same rule to your bras – you have to think a few sizes bigger, especially since you might use nursing pads: they take up extra room.

**9** Prepare some shirts that you do not mind staining with leaking milk (Uh, gross, but what can you do?).

**10** Consider buying a breastfeeding pillow WITH back support (try a few and see which one works best for you) or a nice nursing chair. Also, stock up on Crystal light or your favorite beverage, my friends – once you start breastfeeding, you'll be so thirsty, it is as if you got stuck in a desert!

My mother groaned! My father wept.
Into the dangerous world I leapt:
Helpless, naked, piping loud:
Like a fiend hid in a cloud.

Struggling in my father's hands,
Striving against my swaddling-bands,
Bound and weary I thought best
To sulk upon my mother's breast.

William Blake, *Infant Sorrow*

*33*

# BECOME A LIONESS

## *(and fight common sabotages in the hospital-jungle)!*

You just gave birth. You hear the baby's cry, see a scrunched-up little face, and count ten fingers and ten toes. There is a moment of euphoria and relief. Then suddenly, the exhaustion overwhelms you. You feel like an animal in a jungle, surrounded by strange noises and smells. You remain in the wet hospital gown, with iodine that burns your skin and stitches that itch. Part of you wants to take a shower, sleep, and eat – do everything human. But the other part of you wants to finally see and touch the baby who was hidden inside of you for nine months. At precisely this point, the hospital staff routinely yells orders to get you on another stretcher and out of the room, because they have to prepare for the next delivery. They tell you that you can spend more time with your baby later.

You have just survived labor and delivery; you look wild and untamed; somebody is now in your way. This is the time to turn into a lioness, to fight for the right to be with your baby. During the next few days, you will realize that much sabotage exists in the hospital-jungle. Therefore, it is helpful to know what lies before you and prepare the best combat strategy (although we promise it is less brutal out there than it sounds). You don't always get help in hospitals. It can be very frightening. But if you come with the heart of a lioness and the soul of a mother, you and your baby will make it through.

**After an uncomplicated delivery, hospital staff makes statements such as: "You can try to feed your baby later! We need to get you transferred."**

$\mathcal{T}$hough spending the first few moments with your baby is not life-saving, it may be life-altering, the beginning of a special bond between the two of you. The extraordinary moment of holding your baby for the first time should not be rushed. Data has shown that early skin-to-skin contact (placing the baby on his stomach on the mother's bare chest at birth or soon afterwards) has positive correlations with breastfeeding duration, maintenance of infant temperature, infant blood glucose, and maternal well-being.[7] When the baby latches, the mother provides colostrum that coats the baby's stomach, prevents intestinal problems, and increases immunity (never mind that it stains your shirt bright yellow).

AN IMPORTANT CAVEAT: If there are medical complications related to your delivery, or you have just come out after a C/S, breastfeeding can wait. If your baby is critically ill and cannot take food by mouth, you can pump the colostrum in order to save it for later use.

## SABOTAGE SOLUTION:

Explain that the American Academy of Pediatrics advises placing the baby on the mother's skin right after birth to encourage breastfeeding; the American College of Obstetricians and Gynecologists promotes the same idea. Tell hospital staff that you would like to follow the most current practice guidelines.

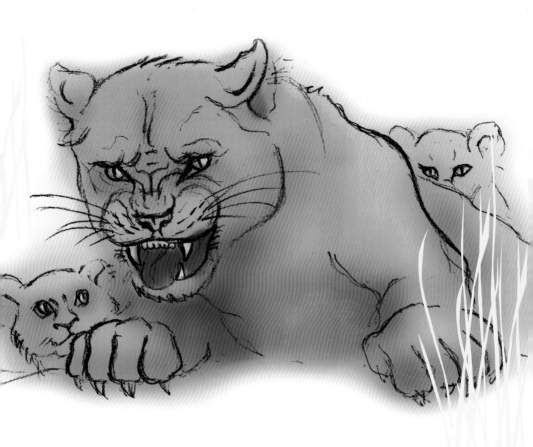

## The Life of a Lioness:

Lions live in a community called a **pride**. The female group is comprised mostly of relatives who stay together for life. The male group includes one or two lions who guard the territory and may only stay a few years, before moving onto another pride. When a lioness is ready to give birth, she finds a hidden enclave. After she delivers, she remains with her newborns for about four to eight weeks, protecting them from predators and nursing them at least eight hours every day. When they are strong enough, she brings them back to the pride.

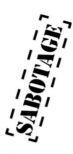**SABOTAGE**

**Hospital staff gives "first-feeds" of formula, instead of bringing the baby to the mother or at least asking her permission. Women who initiate formula-feeding are much more likely to stop breastfeeding altogether than women who exclusively breastfeed.**

Whether the mother and her baby get a chance to spend a few moments together, many hospitals routinely separate them shortly after delivery. The baby is whisked off to the well-baby nursery, where she is cleaned, examined, and observed by medical staff. Hours may pass before the baby is returned to the mother. During that interval, it is not uncommon for some hospital staff to give babies first feeds of formula without consultation with the mother or without a true medical indication. Sometimes, the baby's blood sugar is dangerously low and formula raises it to a safe level. Even in that case, there is usually no need for repeated bottles of formula.

A breastfeeding mother (lioness) tries not to lose sight of her baby for long in the hospital-jungle (or at least assigns the alpha male father to the task while she gets some rest). The father of the baby or other relatives should repeatedly warn all hospital staff about the mother's desire for exclusive breastfeeding. Choosing to have the baby room-in offers maximal protection. Luckily, even if formula has been given, it is possible to start exclusively breastfeeding from that point forward. It just might take a little extra effort (and the lactation consultant) for both the mother and baby to readjust.

## SABOTAGE SOLUTION:

1. Place a "NO FORMULA -- BREASTFEEDING ONLY!" sign on the baby's bassinet (it is kind of like marking a limb before surgery, even though a mistake has less grave consequences in the case of breastfeeding). Once again, there might be justified medical reasons for using formula, but a doctor should inform you and discuss options before the decision is made.

2. Request to room-in with the baby.

3. Remember, formula is not "free": this "gift" potentially costs $1500-$2500 (since once breastfeeding is stopped, you have to buy formula for the rest of the year, not counting the hidden costs of extra doctor visits and missed work days).

## The Life of a Lioness:

A lioness usually gives birth to two to four cubs, but up to nine is possible. The lioness only has four teats, enough to nurse a maximum of four cubs at once. The weakest of a large litter usually get pushed aside and, hence, do not survive. To accommodate several cubs at a time, the lioness makes a great effort to stretch out properly and struggles to avoid sitting on any one of them.

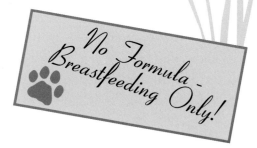

**Your pain may not be taken seriously, or adequately treated.**

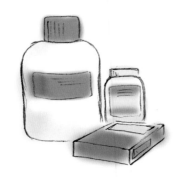

$\mathcal{P}$erhaps, you won two battles in the first few hours after birth: you spent at least a few moments with your baby immediately after delivery, and you got your baby into your room. Now, you see him: he looks like a helpless creature with a tiny mouth that opens hungrily. It seems that nothing could be easier and more natural than to breastfeed him. Yet, when you try it, "natural" feels like a natural disaster: a tornado, or flood. Does the baby have teeth? You scream, and the baby cries; you cry, and the baby screams. Then another shock comes on top of the first one: uterine contractions, which you thought would end with delivery. Now they are caused by nipple stimulation, which releases maternal hormones and helps return the uterus to its pre-pregnancy shape. That's nice to know, except that you are suffering, and nobody seems to offer any help. Postpartum mothers, even after Caesarean section, tend to receive less pain medication than they need to feel comfortable. In lieu of an increased dose, they often get advice about squeezing a little fluid from the breast and spreading it around the nipple and areola. Interestingly, nobody offers such an approach after an appendectomy instead of Morphine. Breastfeeding mothers deserve post-operative pain medications, too. Delivery is actually a surgery, but even hospital staff sometimes forgets that.

## SABOTAGE SOLUTION:

Demand adequate pain medication. Don't be afraid to ask for Tylenol, Codeine, or even Morphine -- these medications are reasonably safe for the majority of breastfeeding mothers. Since a common side effect of these pain medications is constipation, remember to request Colace, a stool softener. This will prevent a lot of pain in the butt.

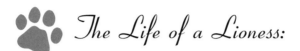

## The Life of a Lioness:

*Interestingly, the lionesses of a pride all give birth around the same time. That way, when one leaves to hunt, other relatives nurse her cubs. So cubs are NEVER left without milk and protection of their relatives.*

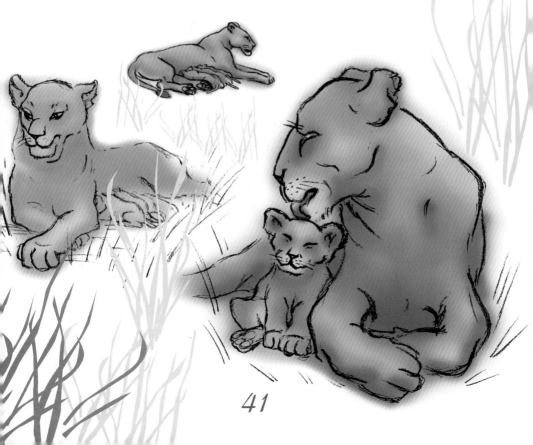

**It is hard to latch: none of the freaking football (or Frisbee, basketball, ping-pong?) breastfeeding positions described in the books work! Nobody knows how to help or seems to be willing to spend time to teach you.**

*O*nce you get your Tylenol (perhaps with codeine) or whatever else you need to feel comfortable, you are now ready to focus on the task at hand, which is latching. The manuals on breastfeeding make it seem simple, with step-by-step descriptions of different positions: the cradle, the cross-cradle, the side-lying hold, and, of course, the football position, which some fathers might get excited about. "Look honey, just hold the baby like a football and move it (referring to the baby) this way!"

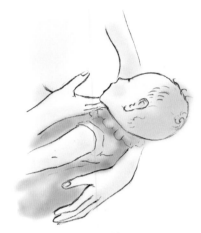

*cross-cradle position*

However, you end up in a "ping-pong position," meaning that you go back and forth between all the breastfeeding positions over and over again. Then, you feel like you are in the ding-dong position: the only person in the world who cannot figure it out. The widespread misconception that breastfeeding is easy is yet another sabotage. When it is surprisingly difficult, some women feel inadequate. In frustration, they cease breastfeeding.

The alternative is to try something that is not mentioned in any of those pretty pink

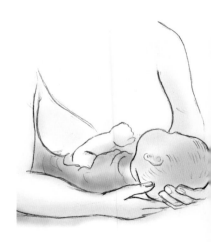

*cradle or cuddle position*

42

nursery pamphlets, a rather crude tactic. Let the baby scream, and when his mouth opens as wide as possible, try to get in as much of the breast that fits. If the baby only grasps the nipple, you take him off the breast and wait for the next scream. This hard-line strategy is worth the extra effort, because it helps prevent cracked nipples. If the baby's tiny mouth manages to make it around most of the areola, you have scored a victory. If you see the baby's cheeks move in and out and hear swallowing noises, it is like striking jackpot: a real lucky break. You know that breastfeeding is working.

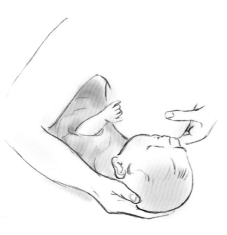

*football or clutch position*

After the baby latches, the next step is to help him breathe: press down on the top of your breast with one finger (your own or your partner's), so that one of the baby's nostrils remains uncovered.

It might take several days of trial and error to realize that you and your baby are the most comfortable in the "cross-cradle" (one of the easier positions) all by yourselves, without any instruction manuals or coaches next to you, thinking it is Super Bowl time. In the interim, do not be afraid that your baby will starve. Newborns are born with enough reserves to survive the first forty-eight hours without any real sustenance, except your and their perseverance.

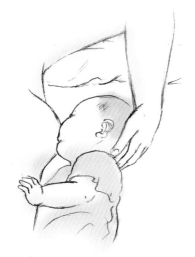

*lying down position*

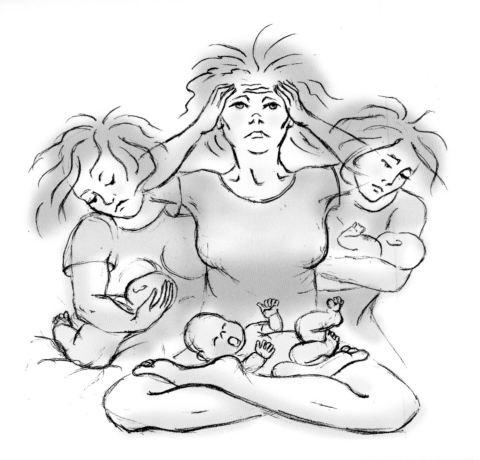

## SABOTAGE SOLUTION:

Keep trying to latch, even if nothing seems to work. Remember, you and your baby will get through this initial hardship. Meanwhile, request a lactation consultant at the earliest possible time!

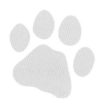

### The Life of a Lioness:

*If a lioness' litter has only one or two cubs, she lets the cubs of her relatives nurse. When her own cubs grow older and start eating meat, she continues to nurse the new offspring of her pride.*

**You are told that your baby is jaundiced, so just supplement with some formula.**

SABOTAGE

In the case of breastfeeding, a lack of knowledge among healthcare providers often spreads misconceptions. One of the top reasons that mothers interrupt breastfeeding is secondary to advice that the baby has jaundice and, hence, they have to switch to formula.

*Jaundice* (yellowing of the skin) occurs in sixty percent of newborns, and it results largely from an excess of bilirubin, the breakdown product of red blood cells. Extremely high levels of bilirubin may result in a condition called *kernicterus,* which is associated with deafness or even the most dreaded complication of brain damage. However, kernicterus is very rare, and the vast majority of babies who have jaundice are at exceedingly low risk. For the most part, it is unnecessary to interrupt breastfeeding. The baby won't stay yellow forever. Half a year later, she might look yellow again, this time around her palms and soles, mainly from eating baby carrots: this is called *keritonemia,* and it is benign.

But we digress from the sabotages at hand now! It is important to understand which types of jaundice exist, and for which types of jaundice it is truly necessary to interrupt breastfeeding.

*45*

# PHYSIOLOGICAL JAUNDICE

Most babies have *physiological jaundice* (in other words, normal jaundice), which occurs between the 2nd to 4th day of life, and disappears by one to two weeks of age. Physiological jaundice occurs because a newborn's liver is not fully developed yet, and thus, there is some delay in quickly eliminating the bilirubin. This slow processing of bilirubin has nothing to do with liver disease. The intestine also participates in eliminating bilirubin. However, newborns have slower intestinal motility than adults and cannot poop out the bilirubin as quickly.

*Supplying more fluid to the baby or supplementing with additional pumped breast milk promotes improved intestinal motility.* Ten years ago, healthcare providers recommended to switch to formula for the treatment of even routine cases of physiological jaundice. Now the center for disease prevention and control (CDC) recommends NOT to interrupt breastfeeding but simply to increase nursing frequency (up to twelve times a day). When hospital staff does not follow current practice guidelines, and advises to switch to formula, even in cases when it is not necessary, they sabotage breastfeeding. (Of course, in severe jaundice, babies may require fluid supplementation and possibly intravenous hydration.)

In addition, light also helps break down bilirubin. This was discovered in a hospital called Floating, which was originally existed on a boat in the Boston Harbor: the babies next to the window never seemed to get kernicterus, while those on the dark side did. In modern

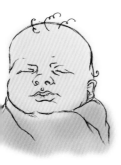

hospitals, the standard care is to use neon-appearing lights above the baby's bassinet, plus little sunglasses to protect their tiny newborn eyes (a bit of the tropics in an otherwise dreary hospital environment). In mild cases, a sunny window still works.

# BREASTMILK JAUNDICE

To make matters more complicated, there is also a rare entity known as *breastmilk jaundice*, which occurs in 1% to 2% of breastfed babies. This type is caused by substances in the mother's breast milk that decrease the liver's ability to excrete bilirubin. Breastmilk jaundice typically starts at 4 to 7 days and normally lasts from 3 to 10 weeks. Statistically, it causes far more concern than kernicterus. The old-school method of dealing with it was to stop breastfeeding and give formula. Some providers remain staunch in those regressive ways. In current practice, it is usually not necessary to stop breastfeeding. The management in most cases simply requires periodic monitoring of the level of bilirubin in the blood, increasing feeds – and yes, placing the baby in a crib next to a sunny window!

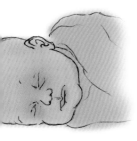

# ABO AND Rh INCOMPATIBILITIES, GALACTOSEMIA, AND OTHER RARE ENTITIES

If high bilirubin appears within the first twenty-four hours, the cause is much more ominous: a major concern is blood group incompatibility, including *ABO incompatibility* and *Rh incompatibility* (when the baby's blood type is different than the mother's, maternal antibodies might act against the baby's blood, causing blood cell damage and excess bilirubin). Treatment may include blood transfusion. The last thing people should worry about in such a critical situation is breastfeeding.

At the same time, if a baby is sick or premature, pumping is definitely an option to consider. A supplement may be added to the breast milk for some needed extra calories. As mentioned previously, breast milk has been shown to reduce the risk of morbidity and mortality in premature babies.

There are also rare causes of jaundice, including one type called *galactosemia* -- an inborn error of metabolism in the baby, in which babies are missing the enzyme that breaks galactose, found in milk, into lactose and glucose. In such cases, breastfeeding should be stopped immediately. However, these actual contraindications are rare.

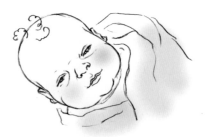

## IN SUMMARY:

The most common hospital scenario is that babies have very mildly elevated level of bilirubin, yet mothers are advised erroneously to formula-feed or supplement with formula. It is important to ask a pediatrician the exact type of jaundice your baby has, discuss it with her, and then make a knowledgeable decision.

## SABOTAGE SOLUTION:

Ask the pediatrician:

1. Does my baby have physiological jaundice, ABO or RH incompatibility, or another rare form of jaundice?
2. Can I just increase the frequency of nursing or pump milk instead of giving formula?
3. Is my baby's level of bilirubin dangerously high?

## The Life of a Lioness:

*A lioness returns from hunting exhausted, and falls asleep. All the cubs, both her own and her relatives', wait for this moment to sneak up on her and nurse to their hearts' content.*

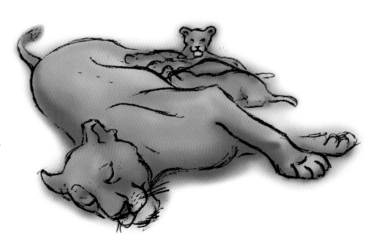

**You have breast engorgement or other problems. The hospital staff often fails to provide you with useful solutions. Instead, they advise you to supplement the baby with some formula until your breastfeeding problem disappears (miraculously).**

SABOTAGE

$S$o what is the big deal about supplementing with formula? It endangers breastfeeding by reducing milk production. After all, the breasts act like a free market, in which demand meets supply. If the baby takes formula, he needs less from the breast, and the breast knows it! On the other hand, if the baby nurses over and over again, the breast gets revved up! Genes get activated; proteins get expressed; and cellular machinery turns on. That's why it is so important to breastfeed for the first several weeks. Those weeks play a major role in determining milk production. After supply has been well established, an occasional formula-feed will have far less of a negative impact.

But even if formula is given in those first few weeks, for whatever reasons, it is relatively simple to increase supply again: increase pumping or feeding frequency, and in just a few days, the body will adjust, responding to demand. A bottle or two of formula won't ruin everything, but bottles add up. You can't trick your breasts or your baby, my fellow sufferers!

Sometimes, in the free market situation, demand exceeds supply, and the market experiences surplus. When your breasts produce temporary surplus, it is called *engorgement*. The breasts feel like water balloons about to pop. Some women think that switching to formula will end their discomfort. One friend described how her breasts felt so weighty and huge that they caused back pain. (O those artists admiring big breasts! Little do they know that pain often accompanies beauty!) The baby couldn't get his little mouth around her breast. No pump was available, or if it was around, nobody bothered to bring it to her. Unfortunately, she had to stop breastfeeding. A little advice could have helped her: pumping before feeding, cold compresses, and pain medication would have probably alleviated her engorgement. Once again, as supply adjusts to demand over the course of a few days, engorgement disappears for the most part on its own.

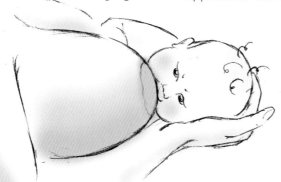

## The Life of a Lioness:

*When they are not nursing or sleeping, cubs play and rough-house with each other. Their mothers, aunts, or grandmothers teach them - in a game - how to hide, find water, hunt, and kill. While the cubs play, the lionesses listen for any approaching danger, in order to guard the cubs from predators.*

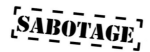

# SABOTAGE

## A lactation consultant mostly is not available.

$\mathcal{M}$ost nurses and pediatricians, if I dare say so myself, do not receive adequate training to provide assistance on how to breastfeed. In addition, for hospital staff, it is sometimes easier and quicker to offer a bottle of formula than to try to get a tiny baby and her crazy postpartum mother to figure things out. Thus, the real contraindication to breastfeeding is not a medical condition, inability to latch, poor milk supply, or nipple problems, but *rather the lack of adequate support and resources.*

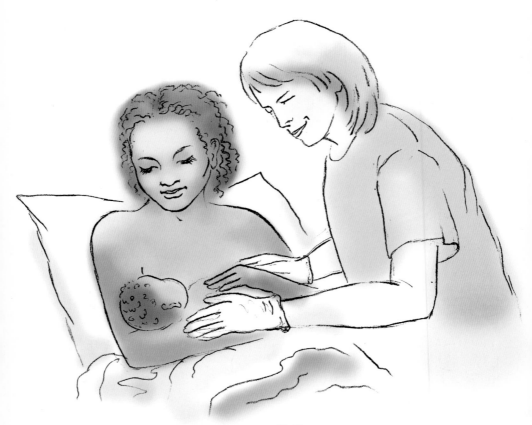

The emphasis in American hospitals revolves around achieving the best possible outcome of a healthy mother and baby. Of course, nothing is more important. But routine preventive care often goes by the wayside. The fast-paced delivery and discharge system in the United States leaves many women, especially those without family support, struggling in the first days of motherhood. Most women say that the hardest part of new motherhood is actually the beginning of breastfeeding (even harder than childbirth).

There are professional lactation consultants at most hospitals that provide much needed assistance. However, sometimes they do not work weekends or evenings, or the hospital only has funding to hire one, who may be overworked. She may not routinely see you, unless you demand it. Do not leave the hospital without her helping you. If you are a mother of twins or multiples, the best approach is to hire an additional private lactation consultant, if at all feasible, for extra sessions in the first few days. Twins are a double-delight (if not double-trouble when they are older) but triple-work!

Fight like a lioness – in other words, keep ringing for the nurse, asking for the doctor, demanding answers and pain medication, and so on! You will get your and your baby's needs met.

## SABOTAGE SOLUTION:

Demand to see a lactation consultant as soon as possible. Demand help from the hospital staff.

# The Life of a Mother (a lactation consultant story):

*I* delivered late Saturday night; they brought me my discharge papers Monday first thing in the morning. I told them that I would not leave without seeing a lactation consultant. She marched in two hours later like a warrior. There I was, trying desperately to get the baby to latch, my shirt half way up, ice packs melting around me, the bed in a scrunch position, and my back twisted. "You are certainly not going to breastfeed in bed!" she said, almost accusingly. In a no-nonsense way, she sent me flying into a chair, and recommended removing my grimy clothes for some "skin to skin" contact between myself and the baby. "It is time to get comfortable," she told me. With great dexterity, she posed me into the perfect position, and placed my now-naked baby in precise alignment; suddenly, my baby latched in the most ferocious and perfect way. Her beautiful cheeks rhythmically puffed in and out, and I could hear happy swallowing. For the first time, the pain from breastfeeding subsided. After a quick break, she scooted the baby on another side, and we repeated the process: skin to skin, rhythmic cheeks, sucking sounds. Finally, my baby finished her first real meal. Both of us lay slumped and sweating, our eyes rolling back with relief. I thought the lactation consultant was a goddess. She had given me a moment of raw paradise, a glimpse into the garden of Adam and Eve. That was the moment one of my

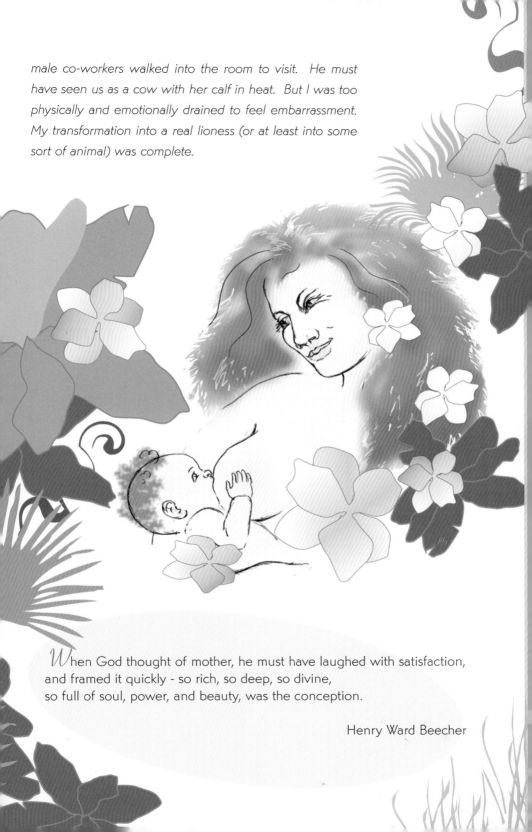

male co-workers walked into the room to visit. He must have seen us as a cow with her calf in heat. But I was too physically and emotionally drained to feel embarrassment. My transformation into a real lioness (or at least into some sort of animal) was complete.

When God thought of mother, he must have laughed with satisfaction, and framed it quickly - so rich, so deep, so divine, so full of soul, power, and beauty, was the conception.

Henry Ward Beecher

# SURVIVE GETTING EATEN UP

## (and solve feeding confusions)!

After you come home from the hospital, it is shocking to realize that you have to take care of this little creature all by yourself. You feel helpless. Besides, you are still bleeding and recovering from surgery. In Russia, Scandinavia, and many European countries, a licensed nurse pays a home visit the

56

next day after hospital discharge and over the first few weeks postpartum. She provides feedback on how you breastfeed, burp the baby, and change the diapers. She even teaches you how to wash the baby and cut the nails (an especially frightening task, unless the baby is deep asleep). In some cases, she might help you around the house.

In the early 1900s, Dr. Josephine Baker, the first woman to earn a doctorate in public health and a champion for children's rights, pioneered a health-care program in New York's lower East Side. It included home visits to all registered newborns by a public health official or nurse. Dr. Josephine Baker proved with data that this type of preventative health program resulted in a considerable reduction in infant mortality. She was so forward-thinking, we are still behind her and behind many countries in the world. Wouldn't it be handy for us new mothers if her ideas had materialized? Or, at least, if we could get some form of help from the father of the baby? Unfortunately, he is off to work right after your delivery, since he most commonly does not get a paid paternity leave.

Left by yourself, you feel confused. For example, you find yourself thinking: which breast should I use now?  Since you have only two, it would seem like your chances of choosing the right one is 50%, but you are still befuddled.  Unfortunately, this isn't Scandinavia or the lower East Side in 1908, my dear.  No nurse will ring your doorbell.

## HERE IS THE BEST REPLACEMENT WE COULD FIND:

| Feeding Confusion | Clarification |
|---|---|
| The one breast versus two breasts per feed debate! | 1) Offer one breast.  The baby eats and eats, then falls asleep.<br>2) Take the baby off the breast, burp the baby, and maybe change a diaper.  Then offer the other breast.<br>3) Repeat in about two hours from the start time. |
| The right versus left breast dilemma (the next feeding) | Start with the breast that the baby took less from during the previous feeding.  (If you forget which breast to start with, it is really not a big deal!  You will use both breasts eventually.) |

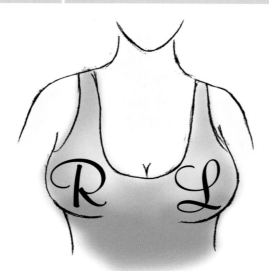

| | |
|---|---|
| Is there a time limit for a nursing session? | It is more like a time goal. It takes at least ten minutes of continuous suckling to empty a breast. |
| True or false: the "never wake a sleeping baby" rule | Unfortunately, that rule does not apply for the first two weeks. It takes a lot of feeds and practice in the beginning, for both you and your baby, to make breastfeeding work. |
| When Enough is Enough? | When the baby cries, it is safe to assume hunger first (then move onto the diaper, and so on). Breast milk is not like Oreo cookies: the baby cannot overindulge! |
| The baby that takes only one side | It is usually a matter of position, not a problem with the breast itself. Keep your baby in whatever position worked on the preferred breast. Do not change the baby's direction. Next move the baby into a mimic position of the preferred breast onto the rejected breast. Voila! |

# But Where is the Milk?

The textbooks say that you should expect mature milk, which looks whiter and thicker, to come after a few days of breastfeeding. They also describe that you get a "let-down" feeling like "pins and needles," and then you know that the mature milk has arrived. However, it is sometimes hard to know when this "let-down" happens. The truth is that you may never feel "let-down," but that does not mean that you are not making enough milk to

59

meet your baby's needs. It can take up to five days for mature milk to arrive, particularly for first-time mothers. Meanwhile, if there is a concern, you could help increase milk supply by applying warm compresses to your breasts and massaging them in a circular motion, working from outside to center. And, of course, if you breastfeed frequently and pump religiously, you speed up the process of mature milk coming in. At some point, you will spurt out fountains of milk more impressive than the Fountain of Trevis in Rome or the Neptune Fountain in Bologna. In the interim, perhaps it is better not to worry about the color or thickness of your milk. The last thing that you need is to spend your time squeezing your breasts and analyzing the drops. There are many other activities to occupy you for the first few weeks with your newborn (the highest rating goes to napping).

### The case of the milk-stained shirt:

*For fresh stains, rinse with cold water ASAP for a few minutes. If the stain remains, blot in some detergent and soak for half an hour (you can rub more detergent in up to every five minutes), then rinse with cold water. If that does not do the trick, try soaking with a stain remover for ten minutes.*

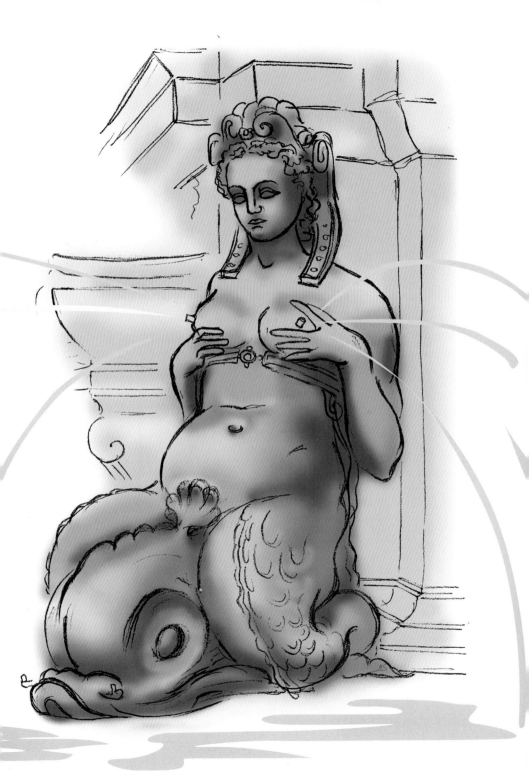

61

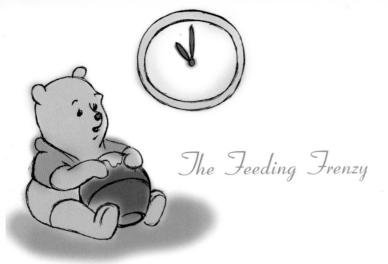

# The Feeding Frenzy

$\mathcal{A}$ normal baby consumes approximately four ounces every four hours. In between, he "sleeps like a baby." Meanwhile, you nap, enjoy a cup of tea, or read the paper. YEAH, right! Real live babies do not wait around on a schedule. Every hour is a big fraction of the baby's life. For newborns, it is always time to feel hungry. They are like Winnie the Pooh, who always feels "eleven o'clockish" (time for a big snack of honey). Some babies eat every fifteen minutes in the first few weeks. One woman friend put it more bluntly: "Those breastfed babies -- they stay glued to the boob!"

### To use a pacifier or to become one?

*A pacifier can interfere with the breastfeeding process. Also, pacifiers can cause dental*

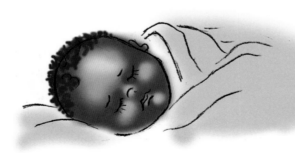

*anomalies. For the first several weeks, you are a much better pacifier, even though you once thought of yourself as a higher-being.*

Many women think that when their babies eat at unbelievably short intervals, looking ravenous and insatiable, something is wrong: women worry that they are either not producing enough milk, or the baby is starving. The reason for the babies to eat so much is three-fold: first, breast milk is more quickly digested than formula; second, newborns need to eat an incredible amount to grow; and third, breastfed babies use the breast as a pacifier. Thus, eating meets both their physiological and psychological needs.

### Other mammals eat less often.

*Rabbits only feed once a day; tree shrews once every two days; a deer leaves its fawn in the woods hidden, and comes to nurse twice a day; a wolf may come to its den to nurse its pups two to three times a day. Why do our babies feed every fifteen minutes?*

The American Academy of Pediatrics has issued a statement against popular baby books that promote early initiation of feeding schedules, instead of feeding on demand. Breastfed newborns whose meals are spaced out hours apart have been known to come to the emergency room in a listless state secondary to dehydration. The recommended amount of feeds in the beginning is between eight to twelve times in a twenty-four hour period (but in reality, some breastfed newborns feed so often that you lose count).

There are exceptions: some babies sleep so much in the beginning that it is necessary to wake them every two to at most three hours to feed (that means two hours after the baby last STARTED eating). Of course, every baby is different, but all breastfed babies require frequent feeds in the first few weeks. Some textbooks talk about differences in babies as though it is reflective of their personalities (lazy feeders, energetic feeders, and so on). Isn't it a bit premature to psychoanalyze characters? They are all little princes and princesses to us mothers.

### The Royal Meal:

*A breastfed baby receives a first and second course meal with every feed. When an infant starts to nurse, he drinks the low-fat foremilk, which satisfies his thirst. As he continues to nurse, he gets the calorie-dense hindmilk, which satisfies his hunger. That is why it is best to let the baby linger on one breast before moving to the next.*

## Then Again, There is the Cluster Feed!

Just when you think that your newborn is eating less often (like only every hour), the clock strikes 5 PM. And then, suddenly newborns get extra fussy. They seem to want to eat and eat and eat even more, beyond your wildest imagination. This is called the cluster feed. Like bears preparing for winter hibernation, newborns are preparing for the few extra hours that they sleep at night (if you are lucky). These nursing sessions are exacting for mothers. It is like running for five miles: you are panting and sweating; you want to collapse; just when you think you are finished, somebody tells you that you only made it half-way. Continuing on is an emotionally and physically grueling process. But take a deep breath. It will get easier soon. Months later, your baby will often take only ten or twenty minutes to eat. And even if the baby takes longer, you will feel relaxed instead of drained. While breastfeeding, you will be catching up on the evening news, watching Netflix movies, or talking on the phone with your friends. You will forget all about the cluster feed, except during the baby's growth spurts when the cluster feed comes back at you (around six weeks, three months, six months of age, and any time in between). But soon enough, your baby will grow up to be a teenager who will cluster feed from the refrigerator!

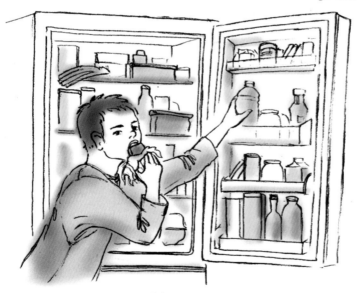

When I am grown to man's estate
I shall be very proud and great,
And tell the other girls and boys
Not to meddle with my toys.

Robert Louis Stevenson, *Looking Forward*

# The Nipple Problems

Most women who continue to breastfeed may experience some nipple or breast problems, from the most common (cracked nipples) to the most severe and dreaded (mastitis, which is a serious infection). These problems require immediate attention. Among the reasons that many women stop breastfeeding is that when problems arise, women do not get professional advice or adequate medical care.

There are relatively simple ways to address some of the most common problems.

## THE NIPPLE HELP GUIDE

| Problems | Descriptions | Tips for Solutions |
|---|---|---|
| Cracked nipples | These occur when the baby takes the nipple instead of the aerola. | 1) When the baby is ready to eat, wait for the baby to open his mouth wide. Then try to get the baby to bypass the nipple and latch onto the areola. If the baby has latched incorrectly, try again (and again).

2) Purified lanolin cream for breastfeeding mothers is like sun block in the tropics — it needs to be applied liberally and often (and it is safe for the baby and mother).

3) Pain medication helps, too, even if it is as simple as Tylenol (the generic acetaminophen is just fine). |

| | | |
|---|---|---|
| Inverted or flat nipples | During breast development, an adhesion of breast tissue pulls in the nipple. | 1) The baby should not latch at the nipple anyway, so it shouldn't really matter if it is inverted.<br><br>2) One method is to pump right BEFORE breastfeeding to draw out the nipple.<br><br>3) There are nipple enhancers and breast shells available with questionable efficacy. |
| Thrushed nipples | A usually harmless candida infection that causes a white overgrowth on your breasts and in the baby's mouth. | Your doctor will prescribe Nystatin ointment for your nipples and Nystatin suspension (1 ml per cheek) for your baby. |

The fledglings have a language
That is all their own,
They lisp in broken syllables
In a high, clear tone.
Each bird learns first a single word
Quite long for a beginner,
But says it very plainly
   "Dinner
      Dinner
         Dinner."

Anna Bird Stewart, *Baby Talk*

# THE BREAST HELP GUIDE

| Problems | Descriptions | Tips for Solutions |
|---|---|---|
| A galactocele | This is a rare complication, when breast milk thickens too much in one acini, causing a milk cyst. | A galactocele usually requires needle aspiration (inserting a fine needle and then drawing out the fluid) by a doctor. |
| Mastitis | A dreaded breast infection that can make the breasts red, swollen, hot, and painful. Mastitis occurs when thickened milk clogs a duct in the breast, and then bacteria gets stuck with no way to travel out.<br><br>In the future, frequent feedings or pumping can help prevent mastitis. | 1) The treatment is to remove the blockage and get the milk to drain forward by nursing and pumping.<br>2) If the pain of breastfeeding is unbearable, pumping in lieu of nursing is an alternative (and the pumped milk is safe to give the baby).<br>3) Hot compresses may also help.<br>4) Antibiotic treatment for the mother is urgent.<br>5) Although it is not a standard recommendation, pain medicine should be requested. |
| A breast abscess | If the infection festers in one spot, an abscess (which is a walled-off collection of fluid) occurs. This is an awful complication, which can usually be prevented with early treatment (see mastitis). | 1) Sometimes, antibiotics are enough, and the abscess drains spontaneously.<br>2) Other times, a needle or even a small incision may be required to get the abscess to drain. |

You only have two eyes, two ears, and two breasts — if one of them looks different from before, or especially hurts, it is best to check promptly with a doctor. Some women report that their complaints are not taken seriously by their healthcare providers. If those people ever experienced similar pain, they would throw every known narcotic in your direction (unless the drug was contraindicated in breastfeeding). They would understand that the pain of an infected breast is no joke. Any ignorance regarding this subject harms women and their babies — and fighting against it helps future breastfeeding mothers.

If all else fails to ease suffering, there is an adjunct technique that might help: **screaming**. People around you should be prepared. They should respond with empathy. They should send you dozens of roses. They should call you Woman of the Year for your courage and perseverance. Alas, nobody recognizes what some nursing mothers endure. Luckily, for most of us, the good parts of breastfeeding certainly outweigh the grisly.

69

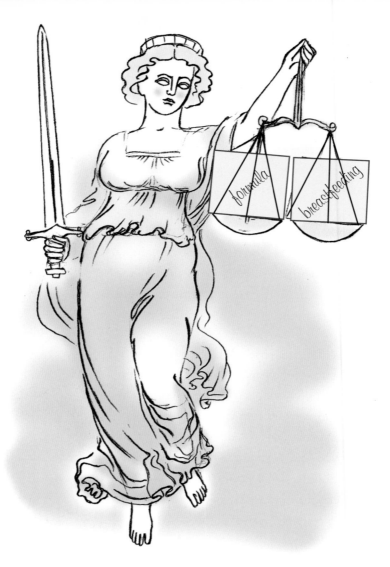

## The Quitting Dilemma

*I*n the interim, breastfeeding can hurt, even without an infection. Many books on the subject cynically gloss past these troubles as "a little soreness at the nipples." Perhaps this is true for some amazon types who run triathlons while pregnant, but not for most of us. It helps to know that it is normal to feel pain and frustration at first. That way you are prepared, at least emotionally. However, it is impossible to know if breastfeeding really works for you without a trial period of six to eight weeks. The first weeks of breastfeeding also offer the greatest benefit to the baby (although, of course, there are continued benefits for the baby if you breastfeed longer).

Formula-feeding brings a different set of concerns. During times when a formula-fed baby is fussy, colicky, or constipated, many mothers worry that something is wrong with the brand that they have chosen. Since there are several types of formula, including cow's milk-derived, soy, and protein-based (the latter ones get more expensive and smelly), families end up changing from one formula to another (even though this is rarely medically indicated). Thus, while breastfeeding invariably gets better and easier, the same cannot be guaranteed for formula-feeding.

Women who decide to bottle-feed may experience a few days or even a week of discomfort from engorged breasts. Ice-packs and a tight bra may provide some relief. Cabbage leaves (raw cabbage) placed in the bra and changed every few hours can help, too (as they do in weaning). Those cabbage leaves also leave a scent in bras that may not disappear after washing.

Many of our mothers used a drug called bromocriptine to stop the flow of breast milk by blocking prolactin (which stimulates milk production). However, bromocriptine is no longer approved for the use because it has been linked to heart attacks and strokes.

The final decision between breastfeeding and formula-feeding should be your own. Nobody should pressure you to continue if you feel miserable. This decision is not about your spouse, cousin, or even the new health campaign that compares SMOKING DURING PREGNANCY to NOT BREASTFEEDING. The government does not provide any considerable help for women, yet launches a surgeon general's health campaign that in effect lays the blame on women for not breastfeeding, stirring up feelings of guilt.

A decision to breastfeed or not to breastfeed is a highly personal decision based on your physiological and mental states. There is more to life and motherhood than breastfeeding, and that is unceasing love, labor, and sacrifice for your baby. If you continue to breastfeed, you should feel good about yourself. If you don't, you should still feel good about yourself. In any case, your love's labor will not be lost — your baby will always need you more than anybody else in the world, not for your breasts but for your heart and soul!

Dance, little baby, dance up high,
Never mind, baby, mother is by;
Crow and caper, caper and crow,
There, little baby, there you go:
Up to the ceiling, down to the ground,
Backwards and forwards, round and round.
Then dance, little baby, and mother shall sing,
With the merry coral, ding, ding, a-ding, ding.

Ann Taylor, *The Baby's Dance*

# REGRESS TO A PRE-SCHOOL LEVEL

*(it is all about pee and poop)!*

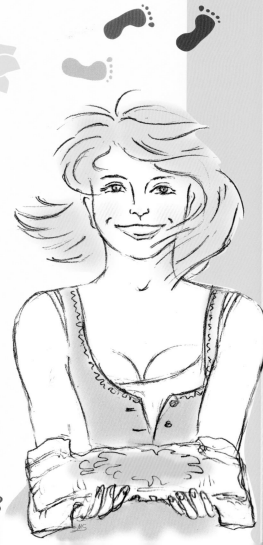

$P$robably, you and your baby have mastered the art of latching, at least sometimes.   Maybe you even figured out what the cross-cradle position means.   Yet, you are facing new challenges.   You are facing (literally and figuratively speaking) diapers filled with pee and poop.   Suddenly, nothing seems to

73

hold your fascination, not even your former hobbies or *Desperate Housewives*. What comes out of your baby seems critically important, if not acclaimed.

Maybe you read Tolstoy's *War and Peace*, or you saw the movie; then you recall lively Natasha Rostova (in the movie played by Audrey Hepburn) coming out of her nursery disheveled, in a dressing gown, proudly displaying to her family a dirty diaper filled with yellow poop, instead of green, as it has been when her baby was ill.

Now, you are just like her. And oh my god, the colors that YOU will see. You may have been your class valedictorian. You may have a Doctorate. You may have earned your way to the top. Now, it is back to the very primitive in life. And yet you feel confused and befuddled.

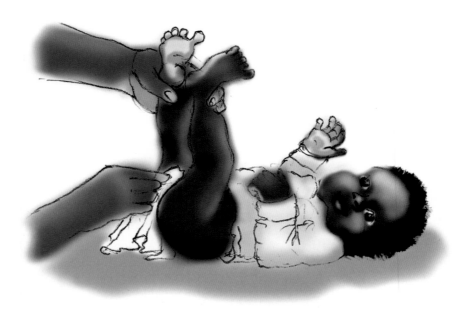

# How do I count again?

You can tell if a baby is hydrated versus dehydrated by the amount of pee and poop. How much is enough? Every baby is different, and there is only a rough guide. It is actually more like a quota. If you meet it, you can breathe sighs of relief (if only you could also sleep). If you exceed it, then you can brag to all your friends about your over-achiever (or at least, you will find yourself oddly tempted).

With pee, there is a simple rule. First, you have to know that there are twenty-four hours in a day. You should expect one pee in the first day, two pees in the second day, three pees in the third day, and so on, until you get above five! Let's review: Do, Re, Me. A, B, C. Pee: 1, 2, 3, 4, 5 (on days 1, 2, 3, 4, 5)! You think you have it down pat, but then you realize you cannot see any pee! Modern diapers absorb everything; you have to feel them in order to know (they weigh more when wet, so break out the kitchen scale).

Now onto poops, which are a bit trickier.

*For the first two days, expect a few (one or two).*
*For the next two days, expect some more (two to four).*
*Around day five, wait a while (and get three to five in a pile).*

This will continue for around four weeks. Then suddenly, anywhere from when the baby turns four to six weeks, he may stop pooping altogether! This can go on for days! You will experience absolute fright. You will pray for poop. You will hold vigil over every diaper. You will hysterically call your pediatrician. She will reassure you that this just corresponds to increased intestinal maturity, that your breastfed baby is absorbing all the nutrients, and that you no longer have to worry about poop all of the time. And you don't need to give prune juice or stick a suppository or anything up the baby's bottom. For many days, you will not believe her, but rest assured, she is telling you the truth. Breastfed babies rarely get constipated. Now you and your baby can, for the most part, go on to thinking about less primitive activities!

It may be helpful to keep a record of pees and poops in the first week. If you are anal enough to continue this laborious process much longer, seek professional help (or reassurance from the pediatrician). If you are too tired to tally every pee and poop, keep your partner occupied for this task. Mine took the job quite seriously: he used Excel and a spread sheet, which he proudly brought to our pediatric visit! Remember, as long as these pees and poops appear in range, you don't have to complete all the paperwork. It doesn't get sent with the preschool application! Nor is it a requirement for a passport or driver's license.

To the right is an example of a simple quota tally sheet, which you can fill in by checking the box. Once you checked off the minimum amount, you can forget about it for the rest of the day: after all, more is OK. If you miss one, don't panic. However, if the baby is not peeing and pooping enough, you have to increase nursing frequency, or better yet, you can also pump and

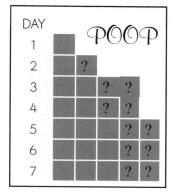

give your baby the breast milk from a bottle (read about the myth of "nipple confusion" later). You could call your pediatrician just to double-check. La Leche league, of course, is another helpful resource.

It is a good idea to follow up with the pediatrician to check the baby's weight and hydration a few days after discharge, then at two weeks, and one month. For the baby's first fifteen months, you will continue seeing your pediatrician more often than your hair stylist. Hopefully, the visits will reassure you that all is well (and you will eventually make it to the beauty salon). If questions arise, it doesn't hurt to make a few phone calls to get them answered. Every mother thinks that she is the only lunatic tying up all the phone lines. The truth is that it is normal to feel confused. We, nursing mothers, are all lunatics tying up the phone lines. Remember, you are still a lioness! So what if someone thinks your questions are silly and repetitive? You are asking on behalf of your baby! And if people are not sympathetic to you and are not prompt with their responses, it is a sign that you should seek pediatric care elsewhere!

# The Color of Madness: You Can't Believe It Until You See It!

*N*ow that you have mastered counting, it is time to learn colors again.

Some people look at poopy diapers with disgust. As a new mother, you look with a genuine interest, and what a bold color range you see (your gorgeous baby made it)!

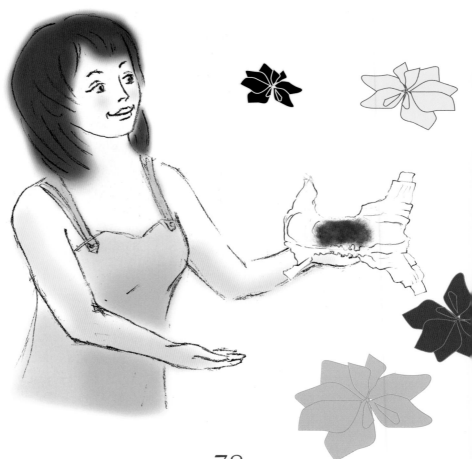

Interestingly, red-green color-blindness is usually inherited on the X chromosome. Females have two X chromosomes (XX), while males have an X and a Y chromosomes (XY). If the gene for color vision in females is not working on one X, chances are it is working on the other X. On the contrary, if the gene for color vision in males is not working on the X chromosome, they are out of luck: since they don't have another X, they have

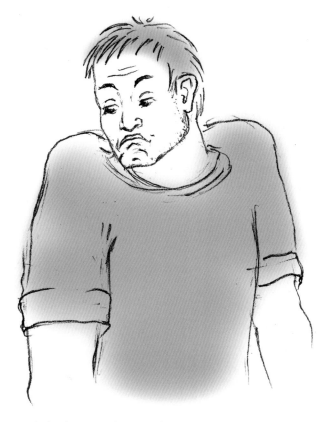

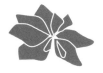

a much higher incidence of color-blindness. Peculiarly, when it comes to the color of the poop, most men appear happily color-blind. They don't seem as fascinated by diapers. For better or worse, the majority of females have preserved color vision.

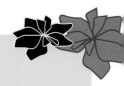

| THE COLOR OF POOP | EXPLANATION |
|---|---|
| It is BLACK like shiny sludge! | The black stuff is newborn poop, scientifically called meconium, which will pass in the first few days. It is what the baby stored in the intestines during your pregnancy (try not to think about how that was in YOUR belly!). |
| It is BROWN-GREEN, and watery! | This is known as the transitional stool, which can appear for several days. It is pretty ugly. So what? We love everything about our baby! |
| It is so YELLOW it fluoresces (plus it is seedy too!). | Breastfed stools are BRIGHT yellow, but they come out surprisingly easily in the wash, and they don't smell like formula stools – a great way to introduce dad to diaper changes! |
| Oh my god, not GREEN again (like Green Eggs and Ham)! | Sometimes, they can be green when the baby is getting too much foremilk (the first part of the feed, rich in carbohydrates) versus hindmilk (the fatty end), but usually this is no big concern. |
| The Red Streak: The Real Scare | Often babies bleed from maternal hormone withdrawal – a little bloody vaginal discharge is normal. Or maybe your baby may have swallowed blood from a cracked nipple. The red streak is probably nothing to worry about, but just double-check with your pediatrician for everybody's sanity (especially if it happens more than once). |
| It's GREYISH or DARKER – and SMELLY! | You have probably introduced solids; this is a good reason for waiting the recommended six months before adding anything beside breast milk. |

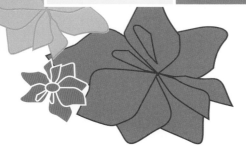

At some point, even you will stop looking and happily let everybody else and their aunt change the diapers. But for the first few weeks, it is your privilege and obsession as a new mother. Thank God, in a few weeks, you will return to normalcy again!

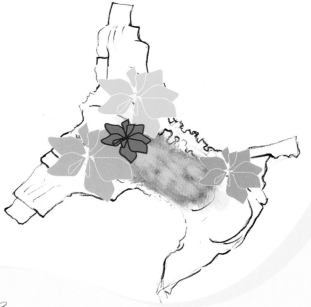

'*Cobalt and umber and ultramarine,*
*Ivory black and emerald green —*
*What shall I paint to give pleasure to you?'*
*'Paint for me somebody utterly new.'*

*'I have painted you tigers in crimson and white.'*
*'The colors were good and you painted aright.'*
*'I have painted the cock and a camel in blue*
*And a panther in purple.' 'You painted them true.*

*'Now mix me a color that nobody knows,*
*And paint me a country where nobody goes.*
*And put in it people a little like you,*
*Watching a unicorn drinking the dew.'*

E. V. Rieu, *The Paint Box*

# SHAPE-UP AT
# BABY BOOT CAMP
## *(the first six weeks postpartum)!*

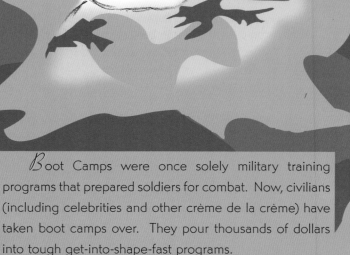

$\mathcal{B}$oot Camps were once solely military training programs that prepared soldiers for combat. Now, civilians (including celebrities and other crème de la crème) have taken boot camps over. They pour thousands of dollars into tough get-into-shape-fast programs.

The first six weeks with a newborn is like a personal Baby Boot Camp, with a few modifications, but free of charge! So call to attention, breastfeeding mothers!

## Baby Boot Camp Instruction

At Boot Camp, there is usually a drill sergeant that barks orders and gets you moving. To your big surprise, the best drill sergeant in the business with the loudest whistle and most intimidating scream has arrived at your home: your baby. He will condition you in no time. The second you fall asleep, he wakes you with a "Ay, ya, YAAYY!" He wants to eat! When you run into the shower, his screams make you to jump out. His diaper needs to be changed! He also makes you hustle to get out of the house. After all, he needs fresh air! Out you go, but before you reach the end of the block, you hear a "YAY!" again. Now, he doesn't want to stay in the stroller; he wants YOU to carry him. Suddenly, you realize that your baby has not only changed but also controls every aspect of your life. Eventually, you will find yourself responding to your baby's needs before he even has a chance to open his little mouth. You have learned to distinguish all of his little desires. You have become an expert **mother.**

# Baby Boot Camp Diet

At Boot Camps, there is commonly a high protein, low-fat diet with strict abstinence from starch and sugar. There are all sorts of other crazy diets around: liquid diets, cabbage soup only diets, calorie counting, starving, Atkins, fat-free, carb-free, raw-foods, and so on. *The breastfeeding diet outweighs them all.* It allows for the return to your pre-pregnancy weight by burning 500 calories a day! Just think: instead of jogging for an hour (445 calories), biking (around 410 calories), or swimming (around 225 calories), you could sit on the couch, watch Oprah, breastfeed, and burn 500 calories extra. What a

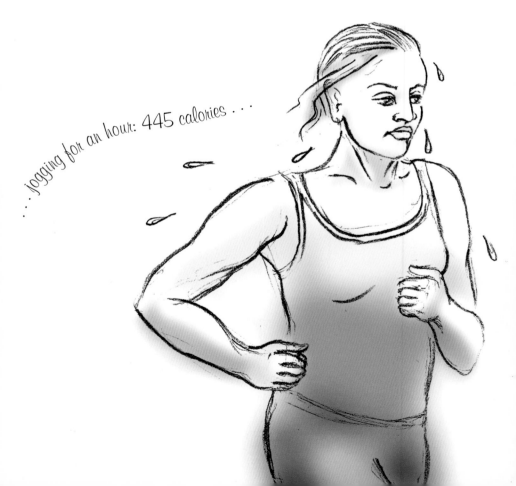

. . . jogging for an hour: 445 calories . . .

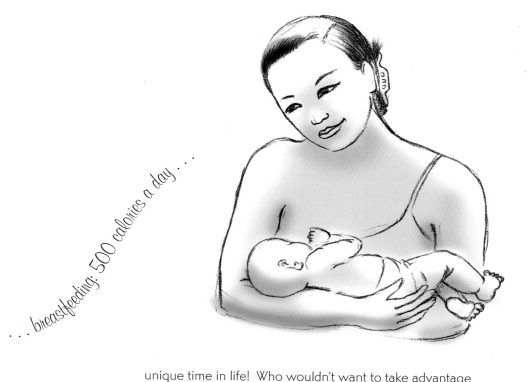

... *breastfeeding: 500 calories a day* ...

unique time in life! Who wouldn't want to take advantage of such an exceedingly rare opportunity in Baby Boot Camp? Any volunteers?

Of course, it is still important to allow time before you expect to return to a resemblance of your former body. As one physician put it: you took nine months to make the baby, so you should give yourself the same time to lose the baby fat!

In fact, in Baby Boot Camp it is imperative to abolish all strict diets in order to maintain milk supply. Starving is *not* an option. After all, milk production increases with body weight, according to studies on sheep, goats, and cows. Of course, the goal is to feel human, but the comparison won't hurt our feelings, right? In Baby Boot Camp, you can lose some weight but not too much. A little ice cream is part of the regimen.

*It is interesting to know that some small animals, like the pygmy shrew, need to double their food consumption and eat five times more than their weight to meet the energy demands of their young. In the case of dogs, puppies demand more and more milk for the first four weeks. At peak lactation, their mothers must consume two to four times above their usual amount. While most humans don't need to go that far, that certainly explains the cravings of nursing mothers for high-calorie foods like milk shakes and fries.*

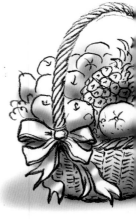

Many mothers are confused about what they can and cannot eat when breastfeeding. A lot of books recommend stringent dietary restrictions for nursing mothers. Broccoli is considered taboo for fear of a gassy baby. Spicy food supposedly causes colic. Chocolate keeps the baby up at night. Nuts are strictly forbidden for fear of an allergic reaction (although there is little evidence that they should be excluded from the mother's diet, unless there is a family history of an allergic reaction). The list is endless.

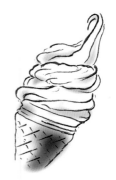

Our breastfeeding counterparts in countries such as India, Japan, and France eat a great variety of foods without such pressure to mind their plates. So why should you give up your favorite things? Very few babies have a real allergy to substances in breast milk, or a milk-protein allergy. When they do, signs include severe discomfort, vomiting, or blood in the stool. Clearly, these symptoms require particular medical attention and often dietary restrictions for the mother. However, most breastfeeding mothers can eat almost any food without a problem.

There are only a few things that need to be avoided religiously: farm-raised and other fish that is high in mercury; unpasteurized cheeses for risk of listeria (but most feta in the supermarket is pasteurized and acceptable, so if you read the label, you can have your Greek salad and eat it too); and raw seafood and meat.

Special dietary recommendations for breastfeeding mothers include drinking eight cups of water or more per day; continuing prenatal vitamins (or hair will fall out in clumps about four months postpartum); and considering a calcium supplement to prevent osteoporosis later in life. The perfect diet includes whole grains, lean meats or other sources of protein, yogurt, and fruits and vegetables. It is also alright to have a morning cup of coffee, Tabasco sauce on your lunch, a decadent desert, and probably even an occasional glass of wine (just wait six weeks post delivery).

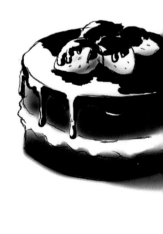

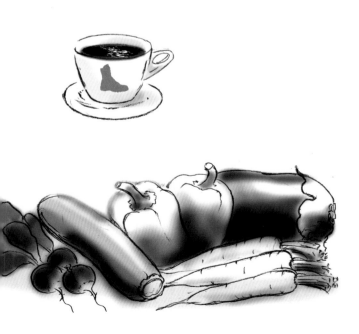

# Baby Boot Camp Fitness

At popular Boot Camps, work-outs include calisthenics, short distance running, weight resistance training, jump rope, crunches, obstacle courses, sports drills, and Pilates.   Alas, general obstetricians routinely advise postpartum mothers to refrain from exercising for at least six weeks.   Most women would not have the energy or time anyway.

Taking care of a newborn is a round-the-clock job. The only slight resemblance to a new mother's schedule is that of a soldier's in combat or a hospital resident's with twenty-four-hour shifts.   New legislation has mandated that residents now have limited hospital hours and the post night-shift day free to recover, after which they are functional again.  If only laws could save new mothers too! They rarely get more than four continuous hours of rest.  Half asleep, they still run errands, lift heavy objects (bulky strollers and car seats), do relay races to fill diaper bags, and keep moving.  All of this can get a mother into shape far faster than any Boot Camp regimen.

On the downside, this schedule can lead to exhaustion and even collapse.   While some popular Boot Camps claim to be tough, in actuality they are forms of vacation. Unlike them, Baby Boot Camp (and maternity leave) is *no* break: instead of focusing on your own body and mind, you become completely responsible for the most important person in the universe: your baby.

This can be very stressful, and **stress is not best for the breast** — it interferes with breastfeeding.  To understand the mechanism, it is important to recall that we have two types of central nervous system responses: the sympathetic nervous system (SNS), referred to as "fight or flight," and the parasympathetic nervous system (PNS), known as "rest and digest." Stress — like in caveman days running from a predator — triggers the SNS, "fight or flight" response. The body shuts down digestive functions and shunts the blood to the heart and legs to race away. The milk reflex is inhibited because of failure of the brain to signal for the release of the hormone oxytocin. Dairy farmers know this — they handle animals at suckling very gently, so that they can "rest and digest" and produce milk.

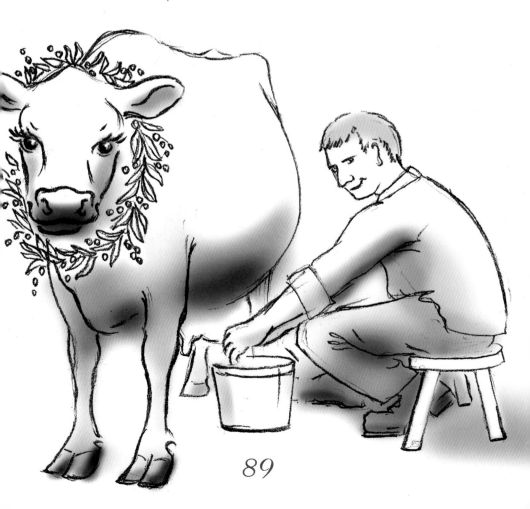

You should be treated even better than a farm animal! The father or other relatives should bring you flowers and chocolate on occasion. They should be washing the dishes, making you breakfast, doing the laundry, cleaning the house, bringing groceries, cooking dinner, and taking the baby on a short walk so that you can nap. It is of medical necessity for everybody around the mother to act sensitive and supportive.

All mothers will feel better by taking care of themselves: napping when the baby does; getting out of the house; strolling through a park or botanical garden with the baby; meeting other new mothers; or simply sitting at an outdoor café with a decaf vanilla latte.

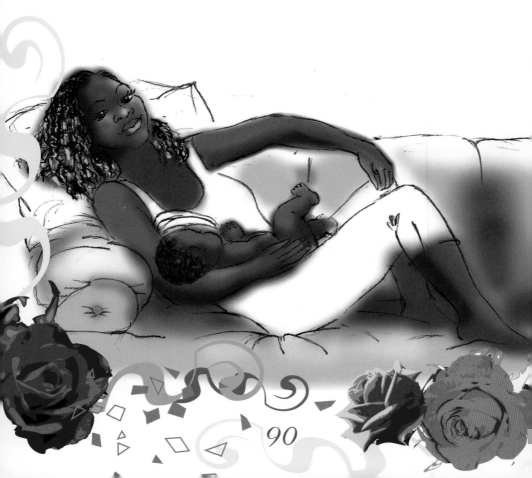

Unfortunately, it is better to avoid large gatherings or crowds, since there is concern about exposing the baby to people (and all of their runny noses)! Any baby who gets a fever (100.4 or higher rectally) before six to eight weeks of age requires a sepsis work-up, which often includes a spinal tap and admission to the hospital for two days. It doesn't matter if the cause is a sniffle, because it is impossible to distinguish a clinically innocent infection from a serious one. So the hope is that if you keep your baby away from people, she will not get sick at all. That is why you rarely meet pediatricians with newborns in crowds.

Even though you may not go out as much, evenings at home can be enjoyable and relaxing with the help of take-out and some good movies. We suggest three top comedies to rent:

1) **Some Like It Hot** (first on the list of the best comedies ever made): starring Tony Curtis and Jack Lemmon, two unemployed musicians who, escaping from mobsters, dress up as women and get a job in an all-girl jazz band. Curtis' gal falls in love with the lead singer Sugar (unsurpassable Marilyn Monroe!); Lemmon's gal gets a proposal from a millionaire.

2) **Tootsie**: featuring Dustin Hoffman, playing an out of work actor who disguises himself as a woman, calls himself Dorothy, and gets a soap opera role. He falls in love with the leading female star, Julie (Jessica Lange).

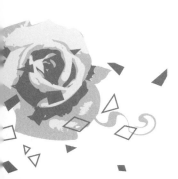

Julie's father falls in love with and proposes to Dorothy.

3) **Les Compères** ("The Accomplices"): a French comedy about two men (Gérard Depardieu and Pierre Richard) looking for a run-away boy, each believing he is the boy's father. Before the boy returns home to his real father, he realizes it is very convenient to have three devoted dads competing for his attention.

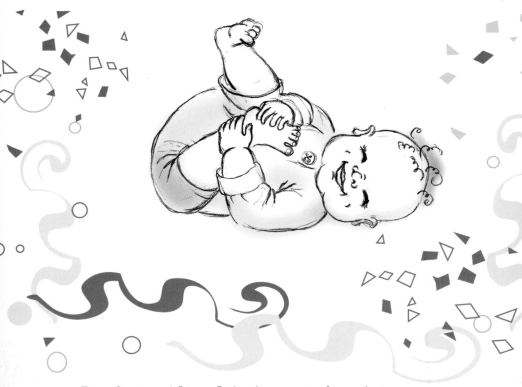

Tony Curtis and Pierre Richard are pretty funny, but there is no better comedian in the world than your baby: the range of noises, facial expressions, and kicks will have you in stitches!

When the voices of children are heard on the green
And laughing is heard on the hill,
My heart is at rest within my breast
And everything else is still.

"Then come home, my children, the sun is gone down
And the dews of night arise;
Come, come, leave off play, and let us away
Till the morning appears in the skies."

"No, no, let us play, for it is yet day
And we cannot go to sleep;
Besides, in the sky the little birds fly
And the hills are all covered with sheep."

"Well, well, go and play till the light fades away
And then go home to bed."
The little ones leaped and shouted and laughed
And all the hills echoed.

William Blake, *Nurse's Song*

# When Nothing Helps: The Postpartum Blues

The postpartum blues are often mentioned lightly, but they are no joke. Nobody gets through the first several weeks postpartum without some tears and emotional and physical fatigue.

Mothers who feel particularly overwhelmed, sad, or withdrawn from their babies are likely experiencing postpartum depression — a common medical condition that is greatly under-diagnosed, even though it is treatable. Prescription antidepressants help mothers suffering from postpartum depression get better and feel like themselves again. With professional help, mothers and their babies get the chance to enjoy each other, as it was meant to be.

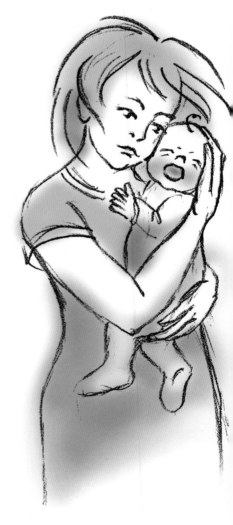

# What Maternal Baby Bonding Is Really All About

*N*o matter how hard the postpartum period was for me, there was one thing that invariably made it worthwhile: my beautiful little baby. I had always read about maternal baby bonding, but the phrase sounded vague. Then, I discovered what that bonding was all about. It turned out that my baby clearly preferred me above everybody else. When my mother, husband, or a friend picked her up, she might look at them for a moment, and then her little lip would curl under, her face would scrunch up, and she would scream. Then, I would swoop her up in my arms, and within seconds, she would rub her little face into my chest and coo with contentment. It was hard not to do a victory dance every time she clearly recognized me and wanted me more than anybody else in her little world. Her special preference for me certainly helped lift my spirits in those first difficult weeks.

*When my clothes did not quite fit yet –*
*And I had not showered –*
*My hair was a mess –*
*I was exhausted, and in pain –*
*Days and nights were mixed-up –*
*It felt good to know that my baby loved me*
*And oh how I loved her!*
*And after she ate, she snuggled into me*
*In such a satisfied and sweet way,*
*With her lips curled into a smile,*
*And those big round adorable cheeks*
*Pressed against me . . .*
*Oh, the cheeks!!!*

It felt good when I took her to the pediatrician, and she was growing beautifully, and I realized that I had fed her, nursed her, and given her the love that she needed to thrive.

And one Sunday, almost two months later, she took a long nap. While my husband watched her, I went jogging; took a nice hot shower; put on a new top and skirt (dresses are hard to wear when breastfeeding); and even read the paper while having tea. Motherhood felt good; and I felt whole again. Yes, it starts out rough but gets better. Later, you will feel like yourself again, only a stronger and more complete version. You might just as well have stepped out of that painting – *Mother and Child* – you and your baby form a complete picture in life (and the father can take it!).

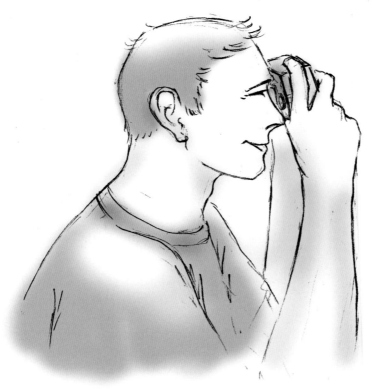

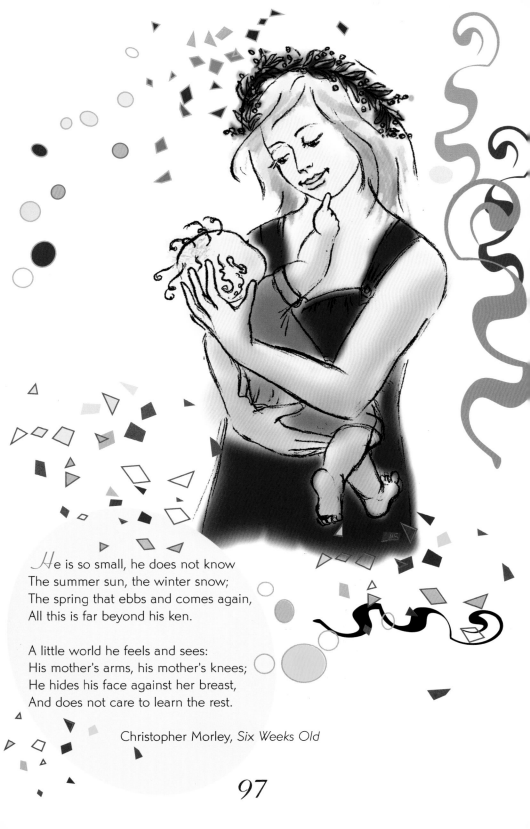

He is so small, he does not know
The summer sun, the winter snow;
The spring that ebbs and comes again,
All this is far beyond his ken.

A little world he feels and sees:
His mother's arms, his mother's knees;
He hides his face against her breast,
And does not care to learn the rest.

Christopher Morley, *Six Weeks Old*

# STRUT YOUR STUFF

## *(in the face of the general public)!*

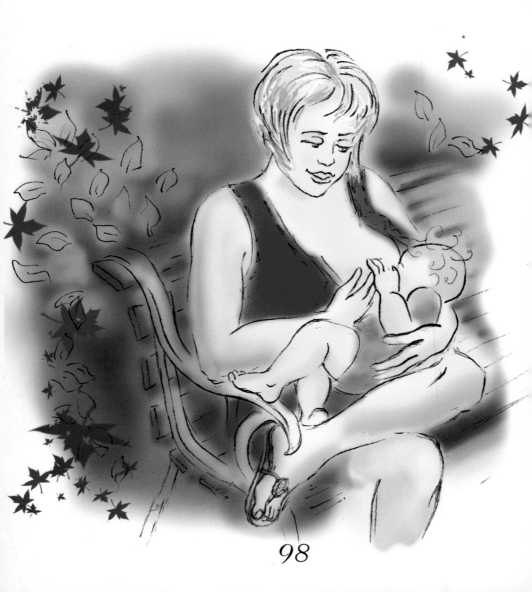

Little by little, life with a baby starts to get very fun. The baby smiles; plays with toys; makes funny expressions; and teaches you new words (Tata, ah-gooooo, ha-daaaaaaaaaaa). One day, she laughs, and you want to tape-record the sound: it is the most joyful music in the world. You are on cloud nine. At night, when the baby wakes up, you feed her half-asleep.

Now you can breastfeed and read; talk on the phone; walk around; sit in a nice chair and relax; or pat the baby's head and play with her toes. Breastfeeding gives you some moments of complete peace and quiet, time to enjoy yourself and your baby. It becomes routine, a natural part of your life. You forget that it was ever hard. You can't imagine how you ever lived without your precious baby. And it is only with her that you feel complete.

Now that you are a little more rested, you can enjoy dressing her up and showing her the world (and showing the world the most beautiful baby that it has ever seen).

The first time you and your baby go out to a real place is an exciting experience, but invariably you forget to put one of the most important things in the big, clumsy diaper bag, such as the diapers.

Some other items that are commonly forgotten include the wipes, a plastic bag to throw away dirty diapers, the changing pad, a toy, a change of clothes for the baby, sunscreen, a hat, hand sterilizer for you after the diaper change, and the baby's blanket.

You end up rushing back home. Or maybe the baby seems fussy, or it rains. The preparation takes longer than the shopping trip or stroll around the park. Then you go out a few more times. The weeks pass. Suddenly, at around two months, you get the hang of everything. The diaper bag gets stocked easily. You quickly dress the baby and go out.

Remember those mothers sitting in parks or cafes, feeding their babies as though it was the simplest and most natural thing in the world? Remember how wistfully you looked at them, feeling you could never be one of them? Now, you *are* one of them. You are sipping ice-tea and talking with some newfound friends. The baby gets hungry, and without even blinking, you feed the baby.

When you breastfeed in public, many people pass you by smiling. "What a pretty sight," they say. It is an endearing image of motherhood, in their eyes, and more importantly, in your own heart.

Of course, there are the naysayers, full of prude thoughts, who advise you to feed the baby in the bathroom (is that where they eat their lunch?); or the immature middle-school types who gawk when you take out your breast; or the squeamish types who cover their young children's eyes, lest they see a part of the human body and the way that a baby eats. . Reactions range from friendly to aggressive. Many of us have heard the story of a Vermont mother who was kicked out of an airplane, because she refused to cover her breastfeeding baby. One would think that fellow passengers would worry more about seeing terrorists than breasts. Many women say that before they had their babies, they cared far more about other people's opinions. Maybe they were too shy to assert themselves. Maybe they didn't like to attract any extra attention. Motherhood changes everything. Life revolves around your baby. In most cases, if people try to get in your way, it is easy to ignore them, but it is even more fun to laugh at them.

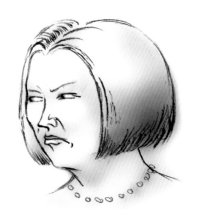

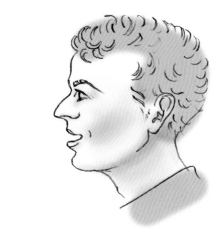

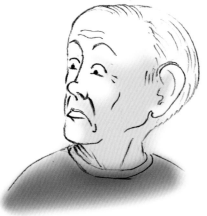

# How to Breastfeed in Public Without Losing Your Sense of Humor

| Type of Public Reacton | Description | A Breastfeeding Mother's Response |
|---|---|---|
| The Prude Dude | He raises eyebrows in shock: he has never seen live breasts and believes that they should be hidden from view, lest they cause too much temptation. | Remember that the stuff on his television screen is much more salacious. He never minded a beer ad, but breast milk is over the edge! |
| The Middle-School Gawker | Although he graduated from the eighth grade thirty years ago, he has never matured past whistling and laughing at the human body. | Shield yourself with your baby's blanket. |
| The Amorous Gazer | He thinks it is beautiful, and wants to look, forgetting that you are a person, not a painting. | Well, you *are* beautiful: it is a nice image. Tilt you head up slightly and pose. |
| The Suggester | She tells you it might be better to go feed your baby in the bathroom or another unappetizing corner. | Act like a Southern Belle, thanking her kindly for the tempting suggestion. Then ignore her. |
| The Comrade | As a fellow mother, she has been through a shared plight and smiles knowingly. Maybe she can't resist giving you a thumbs-up sign. | Smile back: you too will turn into a Comrade eventually. |

## The Fellow Feeder

She needs to feed her baby too! She is happy to have some nice company.

Together, you start a little breastfeeding section in the park. Who needs organized support groups, when you can create them ad hoc?! Breastfeeding is a great way to meet other mothers.

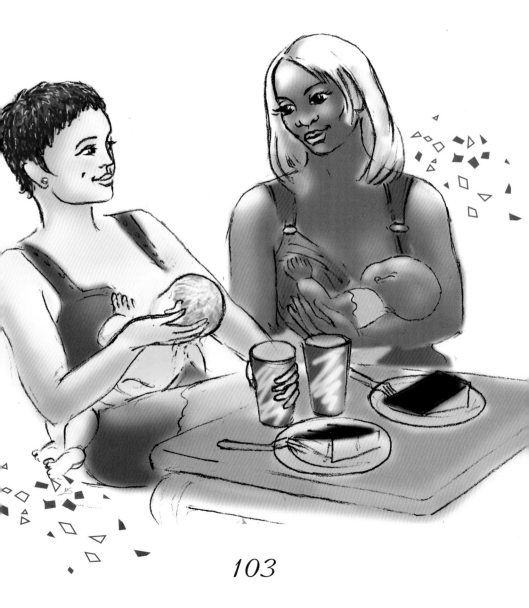

*New Mexico has introduced a new law that protects the right to breastfeed in public. Now mothers can nurse comfortably in shops, cafes, restaurants, airports, train stations, and malls. If evil-doers ask mothers to nurse in the bathroom, mothers can tell them to get out of New Mexico. Let's hope that other states follow suit. Vote breastfeeding!*

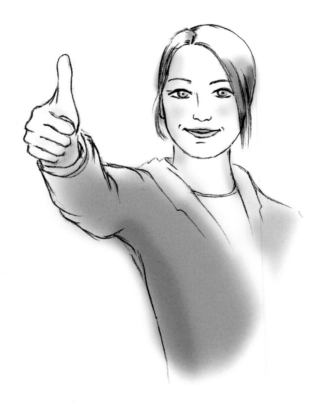

# The HER-story of Breastfeeding

It is surprising that breastfeeding in public is not more widely and openly accepted. Since biblical times, babies were breastfed, including Moses, Isaac, and Rebecca. Virgin Mary nursed baby Jesus. Aside from the bible, written historical accounts omit details regarding breastfeeding in public. *A History of Women in the West,* a comprehensive historical account of the private and public life of women, does not include any description of breastfeeding. However, artists – from Ancient Rome to Medieval to Renaissance to modern times – depicted women in paintings and sculptures, from all classes and walks of life, nursing their babies. These women didn't cover themselves with blankets in shame.

From the artist's point of view, the image of a mother breastfeeding her newborn represents beauty, purity, and simplicity. However, from a historical perspective, the inner world of breastfeeding has always been complex and even cruel.

Women from the upper echelons of society, from Ancient Greece to nineteenth century Europe, tended to avoid breastfeeding. After all, breastfeeding was regarded as the job of low-class women. Breastfeeding potentially interfered with a lady's social life or even image. For instance, it was fashionable among aristocratic Renaissance women to have high, firm, and small breasts, and since breastfeeding could purportedly make them sag or engorge, it had to be strictly avoided. Finally, breastfeeding interfered with marital life. Doctors and midwives falsely believed that sex was harmful to the breastfeeding mother and her baby. You could just picture a Renaissance velvet-capped husband begging his low-bosomed wife to come with him to bed instead of breastfeeding.

*In Spartan Greece, rich women had slaves or poor country women who breastfed for them. However, there was one exception. The law required that a mother always breastfeed her eldest son, the heir. It was thought that there were special advantages to mother-specific infant feeding. Only the most valued babies inherited the right.*

In most societies, for many reasons — whether for the sake of convention, convenience, fashion, or domestic harmony — the rich hired wet nurses. The cruelty lies in that these poorer women often had to neglect their own children and families in order to prioritize the milk-needs of their charges. Alternatively, some aristocrats actually sent their newborns away to wet nurses in the countryside, where in impoverished conditions, some infants died. It is hard to believe, but both poor and rich babies suffered from the breastfeeding customs of the times.

*In Shakespeare's **Romeo and Juliet**, the comic, sharp-tongued Nurse breastfed Juliet, not her mother Lady Capulet. Interestingly enough, Juliet had a bond to her Nurse that was closer than that to her mother. After all, it was to Nurse that Juliet confided about her love for Romeo.*

*Hidden in the tragedy of Romeo and Juliet is yet another sad story. The nurse's own baby-girl Susan was born at the same time as Juliet, but died soon after. Usually, mothers who feed twins or multiples have ample milk (demand meets supply). However, if a woman cannot tend to one child regularly, that is a different story. Was Susan's death the result of forced neglect?*

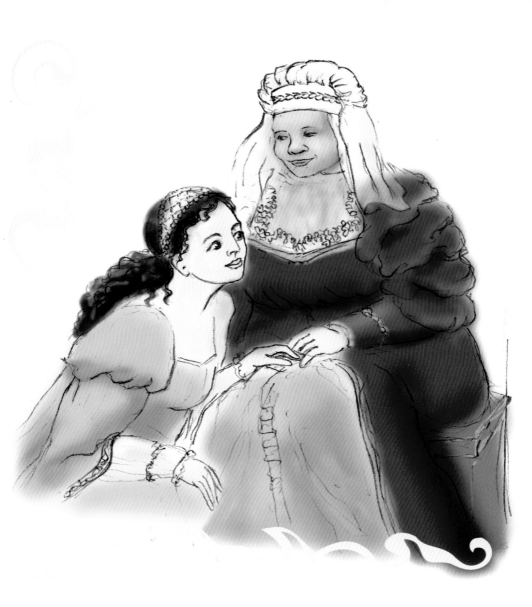

Of course, wet nurses were not always luxuries but sometimes necessities in cases when the biological mother died at childbirth, or she was unable to nurse her child. Since there were no formulas or real alternatives to breast milk, a wet nurse often made the difference between life and death. Some poor families, who could not afford a wet nurse, tried home concoctions, which often led to fatalities in the era before Pasteur invented "pasteurization" (1860).

In 1867, following pasteurization, something revolutionary happened. The distinguished German chemist Justus von Liebig invented the "dry nurse," the first commercial infant formula, known as Liebig's Soluble Food for Babies. Other formulas followed the LIE-BIG! substance in rapid succession. Companies advertised their formulas as better than natural, the perfectly engineered and designed solution to infant nourishment. By the end of War World II, there was an enormous national shift from breastfeeding to formula-feeding. By the 1970s, 75% of babies in the United States were fed on commercially produced formulas, from Nestlé's Good Start to Similac to Enfamil.

Today, breastfeeding rates have remained low, although there is considerable variability nationally. The "top-breast" states are California, Montana, and Washington. The "bottom-breast" states are Alabama, Louisiana, and Mississippi. In Santa Clara, California, over 90% of women initiate breastfeeding; in Laurel, Mississippi, only about 50% of women do. Single mothers, women with only high-school education, and African-American women have lower rates of breastfeeding than married women, college graduates, and white, Hispanic, and Asian women. Due to disparities in education, maternity leaves, and services, there is a shocking socio-economic and racial inequality in breastfeeding. While in olden times, rich women hired wet-nurses, paradoxically, in modern times, poor women end up with dry-nurses.

Breastfeeding has somehow turned into a luxury in the United States, like health clubs, organic food, and eco-travel. How did it become a privilege? The story of breastfeeding remains as complex in modern times as it was historically.

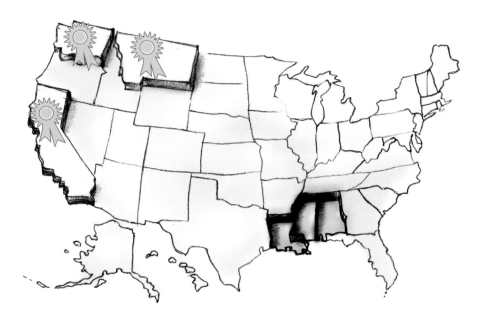

In many countries, such as India, Russia, or Latin America, breastfeeding rates have remained high without striking class divisions. Sadly, this has begun changing, with increased formula campaigns and shorter maternity leaves.

Recently, in the Philippines, around four thousand mothers broke the Guinness world record for simultaneous breastfeeding. They acted in protest against the aggressive marketing of formula.

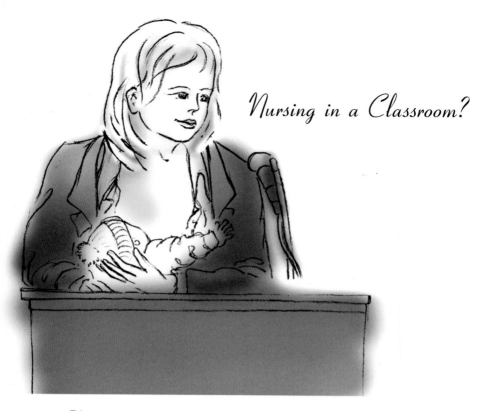

# Nursing in a Classroom?

$\mathcal{D}$uring my fellowship in genetics, I taught a genetics class in the evenings, together with a few other doctors and a genetic counselor. The genetic counselor began to teach the class when her baby was just a few weeks old. She brought her baby to every session. Sometimes, the baby cried, and while she instructed, she calmly breastfed. Her grace and unfledged concentration were astounding. At one point, she started to breastfeed while reading, without skipping a single line. At first, some students raised eyebrows, but soon they became accustomed to it. The next year, her baby turned one-year-old; by that time, I had my baby. I remembered the genetic counselor's previous composure in the room, and told her how impressed I was. "I'm glad it looked that way," she said, "It was so hard. I thought that I was falling apart!" Now, it was my turn to bring my baby to class. In one of the classes, the genetic counselors were learning how to perform a physical examination. At that moment, my baby started crying. In my opinion, my baby suffered enough, since I had to leave her for work during the day. When it was evening, I wanted to make her life as easy as possible. I decided that the precedent had already been set. So, what did I do? I breastfed in front of my supervisor, colleagues, and twenty surprised new students! I decided that I should not feel ashamed of a natural food source! A breast; a bottle; a plate — it is all the same at the end. It was more important for me to provide my baby with food than to care about other people's opinions. Besides, the genetic counselor assured me that it was good for the students to see breastfeeding in order to get accustomed to pediatric visits. "They might as well experience the shock of seeing it for the first time in class rather than in clinic. They need to get used to it. You are doing the general public a favor," she said. Before motherhood, I was certainly not the type to provide shock value. But now, everything had changed — it was not about my feelings; it was no longer just about me: my baby came first.


$\mathcal{H}$ow many days has my baby to play?
Saturday, Sunday, Monday,
Tuesday, Wednesday, Thursday, Friday,
Saturday, Sunday, Monday.
Hop away, skip away,
My baby wants to play;
My baby wants to play every day.

Traditional, *How many days has my baby to play?*

# Special Circumstances When It Helps to Breastfeed

| After shots | Consider giving a dose of acetaminophen right before shots, which will decrease the pain from muscle inflammation and help reduce the chance of fever. Breastfeed right after the shot. When you come home, giving the baby a warm bath and massaging the thighs will also help decrease pain. |
| --- | --- |

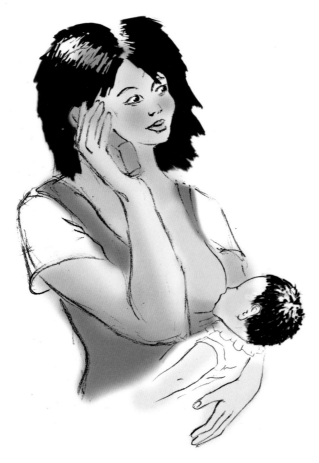

| | |
|---|---|
| On the airplane | Feeding the baby on ascent and descent helps prevent ear pain, which arises from changes in air pressure (when the baby swallows, the pressure in her ears equalizes). A bottle could also work. |
| In a snowstorm or if delayed somewhere | There are no concerns that food for the baby will run out! |
| When you want to read the paper, make a phone call, or paint your toe nails | It is amazing how adept you get at multi-tasking while breastfeeding. |
| When you need to cut the baby's nails | The baby concentrates on eating and lets you trick her (another way to cut her nails is when she is sleeping). |

The game for which I really care
The most about, is playing Bear,
Which Papa plays the best of all.

At first he gives a growl-y grunt,
And then he comes around to hunt
Where I am hiding in the hall.

I sometimes scream an awful yell,
Yet why, I really cannot tell,
Because I'm not afraid one mite,

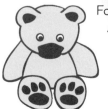

For though he runs me through the yard,
And when he catches, hugs me hard,
I know a Papa Bear won't bite!

Anna Bird Stewart, *Gentle Bear*

# FIGHT THE "YOTTLE' IN YOUR BABY'S BOTTLE

## (with the help of Dr. Seuss)!

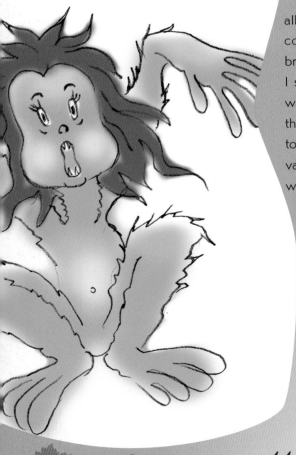

The breastfeeding books all warn mothers about "nipple confusion." They say establish breastfeeding and avoid all bottles. I staunchly followed the advice and waited until week six to introduce the bottle, a month before my return to work (with the help of saved vacation time, my maternity leave was ten weeks).

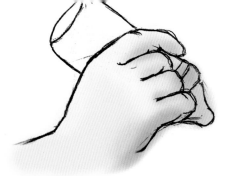

My baby responded to this medical advice about as favorably as she did with her two months shots. She screamed. Her whole face turned absolutely red at the insult. She just wouldn't take a bottle. I counted twenty-seven days left of maternity leave.

The books also advise that the mother should leave the house, and another person, like the father, should give the bottle. My pediatrician confirmed. So did my medical colleagues, who had tried and proven this tactic with several of their own little tykes.

My husband turned into the evil-doer with the dreaded bottle: the baby would have none of it. The poor replacement of pumped

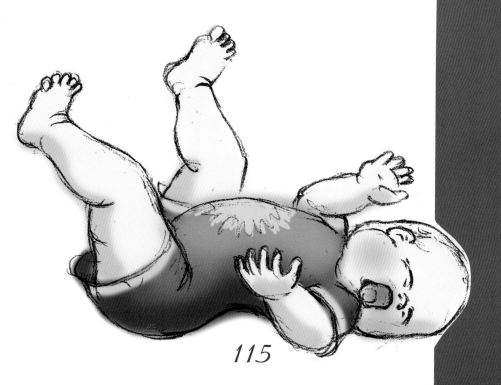

milk did not seem to please her.  She would rather starve than take the bottle.  It was not a good daddy-baby bonding experience.

Maybe she didn't like the bottle nipple?  We tried every nipple on the market, particularly the Aventis and the NUC nipples, which came highly rated by other mothers.  There should be a nipple kit for all the mothers in this predicament, like a variety granola pack!  Our baby

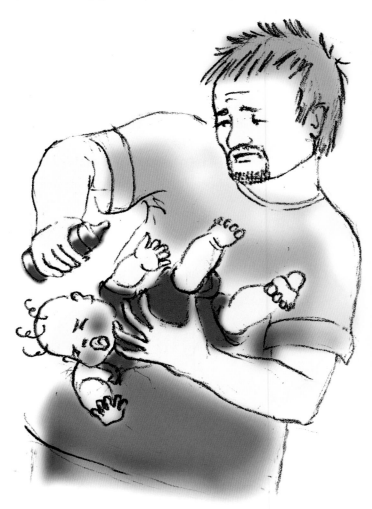

rejected them all. We tried warming the milk, serving it at room temperature, offering it cold, and blowing wishes in its direction. It seemed like we needed some sort of voodoo trick. I even tried the tactic of starting with my breast and slipping in the bottle next. The second my baby felt the artificial nipple tip, she wailed.

That was when I decided my six-week-old had won. After suffering through pre-med classes, making into medical school, completing residency, and finishing the first year of my fellowship, I planned to work as a doctor. But apparently, my baby didn't care for my plans for the bright future, which included taking care of other babies besides her alone. She had her own judgments regarding my priorities in life. So I emailed my fellowship director: could I take some extra leave? My baby won't take a bottle; I could not let her starve. An experienced pediatrician, he kindly responded: "Don't worry. She'll take it eventually." He did not, however, mention changing my return date. What could I do but keep trying; and what did she do but keep refusing? Every other day, I would repeat my e-mail asking to defer my return, and cheerful and encouraging responses filled my in-box: "Hang in there." "Let's wait." "The problem might disappear on its own." All those e-mails about bottles must have convinced my beloved mentor, who is the best doctor I have ever known, that I had gone crazy. Maybe I was not fit to work anyway. The only thing on my mind was breastfeeding or pumping for all those refused bottles. That became my obsession and my specialty.

Two weeks before my return (hopefully, to work and sanity), my mentor kindly offered the following: "Why don't you stop by for just a few hours, and see how it goes." Another doctor in my office suggested that, alternatively, I abandon the house for eight hours, and by the time I came home, the baby would figure it out. "Babies are not going to starve," he said confidently. I certainly was not prepared for a whole day apart, but a morning seemed reasonable. I fed my baby before I arrived to clinic; and I left her with my mother and a bottle of pumped milk in a park just outside the hospital. Within an hour, my pager and cell phone started ringing simultaneously: apparently, it was an emergency. My baby screamed in the background of Bronx sirens and my mother's pleading voice. "Sorry," I said to a room full of doctors, "I have to go!" And I ran out before I had a chance to see their astonished faces.

That was when my second fellowship director got involved in the bottle drama. She told me that she had been through the same ordeal around sixteen years ago, when she had to go back to work, and her son refused a bottle. Luckily, her mother had some advice from the "old country." "Don't struggle when the baby is hungry or upset. When both of you are happy, offer the bottle in the form of play. Make it a toy – babies love to put things in their mouths, after all." That advice worked for her. One of my friends concurred with the principle: her baby took a bottle for the first time while distracted happily with cartoons, even though the American Academy of Pediatrics (AAP) does not recommend television before the age of two. There is a joke that Baby Einstein is so addictive it should be called Baby Crack. Yet another friend said her son took a bottle while looking up at fall trees. Suddenly, there was hope. I too could try games, nature, and even forbidden television without traumatizing myself and my baby!

I spent the next several days of my life with a bottle next to me, offering it every half an hour or so, while singing, pantomiming, and making silly faces. I tried in the park, the stroller, and the car-seat, whenever the baby

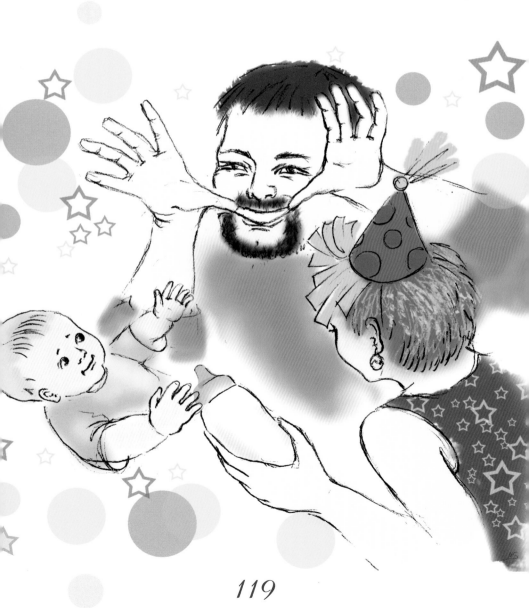

seemed content and happy, but never when she looked upset, or wanted food. And I took the bottle away the second my baby refused it. Sometimes, she took a few sips before turning to a more interesting activity. The day before I had to go to work was Mother's day. My family finished a celebratory luncheon. Afterwards, my baby sat happily in my lap, while I played on the piano songs from *The Sound of Music*. She liked *My Favorite Things*, and started to bang on the piano, too. When I offered her the omnipresent bottle, she suddenly took it: all four ounces. It was her Mother's day present to me. And later that evening, she took another bottle. She learned to take a bottle on her own terms.

The experience made me realize that babies, like most people, don't like the introduction of new concepts when they are upset, hungry, or tired. They need encouragement and comfort to learn; they need songs and soothing voices. Hard-line tactics make everybody miserable. Forget about all the pediatric advice about how to teach babies to take a bottle (although anything will eventually work). Instead, turn to Dr. Seuss: nursery rhymes, happy songs, and silly times. And then your baby won't find a yottle that lives in a bottle after all.

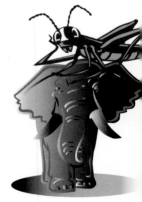

> Way down South, where bananas grow,
> A grasshopper stepped on an elephant's toe.
> The elephant said, with tears in his eyes,
> "Pick on somebody your own size."

A. Nonny Mouse, *Way Down South*

Some women introduced bottles of pumped breast milk from the beginning: their babies never had any "nipple-confusion," and eagerly took either the bottle or breast, whatever was offered first. Other women experienced refusal at the breast. The same tactics of trying whatever the baby refuses, whether breast or bottle, as a form of play works wonders. It takes a combination of persistence, patience, and playfulness. Follow Winnie-the-Pooh's motto: Every day should be festive, filled with gaiety and song-and-dance.

*Tra-la-la, tra-la-la, rum-tum-tiddly,*
*a fly can't bird, but a bird can fly.*

Even for stay-home mothers (certainly the hardest job of all), it is a good idea to introduce a bottle: this is teaching an important survival skill. There is always the fear of an accident, a sudden illness, or a family emergency, which might force temporary separation. You don't want the added worry of your baby crying from hunger. Or on a happy note, maybe you want to leave the baby to jog, get a haircut, or a manicure and pedicure. Or you and your husband plan to go out for an evening (to see that Broadway show and eat at a good restaurant using some of the money you saved by forgoing purchases of formula). After all, you invested so much time and energy on your baby, it only seems reasonable to spend a little time on yourself, too. Just as there is great variety in life, there are many variations to every riddle and rhyme:

*Tra-la-la, tra-la-la, rum- pa-pa-ance,*
*a dance can't girl, but a girl can dance.*
*Tra-la-la, tra-la-la, rump-pa-pa-ish,*
*a fish can't boy, but a boy can fish.*

121

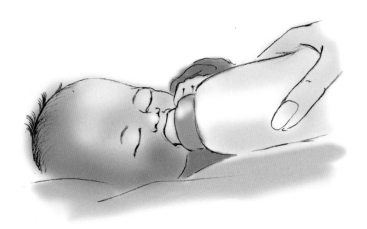

# TIPS TO INTRODUCING A BOTTLE:

| 1 | Consider starting earlier than the common four-six week recommendation - "nipple confusion" is often a myth. |
| 2 | If the baby refuses a bottle, don't push it in the baby's mouth and don't try to force-feed the baby (this will cause trauma and bad associations with the bottle). Move onto another activity and an hour or so later, try offering the bottle again. Of course, breastfeeding should continue as usual. Prepare for hundreds of refusals before succeeding, and don't stress out about it. |
| 3 | If the baby does not like the bottle, do not try when the baby is hungry. I don't know about you, but I certainly don't learn new skills when I'm in a bad mood or starving. A good time to try is half an hour or an hour after the baby takes a nice meal. |
| 4 | Turn to Dr. Seuss: try singing, reading nursery rhymes, and talking in a soothing voice to distract the baby. |

| 5 | Any person and every person can offer the bottle: forget all the rules about only dad offering it. Just make sure the person who offers responds to rejection with a sense of humor. |
|---|---|
| 6 | Try every nipple and temperature in the world, and then realize that whatever you keep offering over and over again will work eventually. |
| 7 | Make the bottle omnipresent. Offer it before sleep, when just awake, outside, while playing, or in the car seat, until the baby decides to play with it and even try it. |
| 8 | If you are not around, try leaving one of your extra smelly shirts for comfort! The baby will instantly calm down when she feels your presence in some way. |

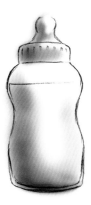

*M*y Mother teaches me at home
To learn my alphabet.
I know it all but W
And that I cannot get.

Do you suppose you could explain
So I'll be sure to see,
Why, when she says, "That's *double you*,"
It isn't *double me*?

Anna Bird Stewart, *Alphabet*

# SLEEP LIKE A BABY

*(or with a baby)!*

The biggest name in the baby world was once Gerber. Now, it is Ferber. Pediatrician Dr. Richard Ferber is the director of the Center for Pediatric Sleep Disorders at Children's Hospital in Boston. In 1985, he published a book entitled *Solve Your Child's Sleep Problems*, where he has set a new paradigm for children's sleep. Dr. Ferber uses appealing terminology — he talks about *comforting* babies through the *learning* process and *teaching* them how to soothe themselves to sleep. It is a lot of words and explanations but it all comes down to one revolutionary idea: *let them cry it out.*

The "cry-it-out" idea has appealed to quite a number of people. As a result, a new word, or term, has been created: *ferberizing.* "Have you ferberized your baby yet?" has become common-vernacular. It sounds a bit frightening to *ferberize* somebody, as if you have given the baby an electric shock.

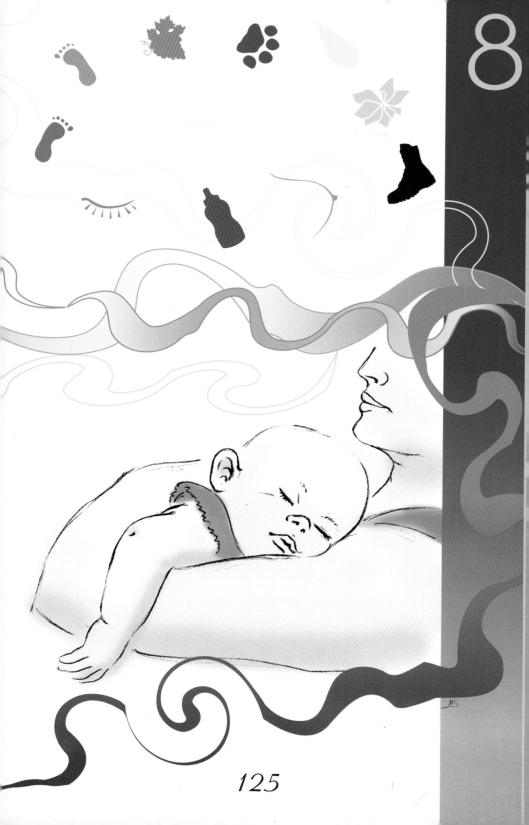

8

125

The process involves initiating a bed-time routine every night at the same time, whether a child is drowsy or awake. You can pat him and reassure him of your love, and then you leave, for longer and longer intervals. He might cry for a while, and you have to let him. You forewarn the neighbors of the medically-endorsed plan so that the police are not called. In a few days, the baby will get used to sleeping on his own and learn to sleep through the night.

Even though Dr. Ferber states that it is unsafe to use his method on newborns, since they can become dehydrated and are not physiologically ready, he claims the process can be started when the baby reaches five months of age.

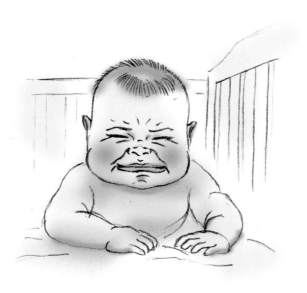

There are rare metabolic conditions in which children cannot safely fast for an entire evening – so let's just hope that these babies never get *ferberized*. Luckily, for the majority of healthy infants, who are exceedingly resilient, the method can be tried without health risks.

The Ferber crowd swears by the method. They claim that after a few hard days, their lives became better than ever. They finally caught up on some sleep, their moods improved, and they stopped bickering with each other. They started exercising again. They became more productive at work. They took back their evenings with wine and guests.

The anti-Ferber crowd tells horror stories about how people pressured them into trying it, and when they finally succumbed, the baby threw up, cried his little eyes out, and the neighbors called the police. The worst part was the guilt.

The choice is left to you: you could let them **cry it out**, or you could tell yourself to **wait it out**.

The *wait it out* side, led by Dr. William Sears, is called "attachment parenting." A warm and bubbly pediatrician, he tells mothers to do whatever feels natural. You can comfort your baby in any way that feels good; you don't have to sleep-train him; you can let him breastfeed to sleep and dream in your arms. Like Dr. Ferber, Dr. Sears mentions putting the baby to bed when the baby feels drowsy. In reality, if you are a devoted attachment-aficionado, you will ultimately end up doing the following: when the baby is really sleepy, you will tiptoe towards her crib, gingerly put her down, and pray that she won't wake up. Sometimes she cries immediately, and then you breastfeed her again, or hold her, or walk around, or sing or pray some more. This approach is kinder and more humane. Unfortunately, for some parents it is just a *tiny bit exhausting*. The baby is rested and happy; you are miserable and grumpy. Motherhood is martyrhood, right?

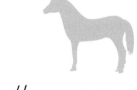

Hushabye, don't you cry,
Go to sleep, little baby;
When you wake, you shall have cake,
And all the pretty little horses,
Black and bay, dapple and gray,
Coach and six white horses.
All the pretty little horses.

American Folk Traditional, *All the Pretty Little Horses*

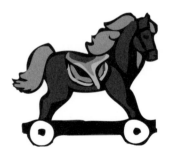

Most breastfeeding mothers are on the highly attached side, especially with their first child. They cannot stand when the baby cries. And so, most of them do something that all the Ferberites frown upon – they **co-sleep** (same room) or even **bed-share** (same bed). You can just picture all the physicians in the best hospital in the country jumping out of the Ferber textbook to point fingers! The downside is that some (but not all!) mothers feel guilty, as if they are doing something against standard American practice. Societal perception is that co-sleeping occurs only in the developing world; but in fact, it is also common practice in many European countries. It turns out that ninety percent of the world co-sleeps and bed-shares. Did Ferber as a baby always sleep in his own separate room? Perhaps his mother might reveal his sleep secrets some day. Maybe she picked him when he cried, without foreshadowing the ferberizing method.

There is more positive view on bed-sharing, which mothers, who could not resist the practice, might find comforting.

Dr. J. J. McKenna, Chair in Anthropology at the University of Notre Dame and Head of the Mother-Baby Behavioral Sleep Lab, believes that babies should never sleep alone (obviously, his ideas are controversial).[8] He points out that mothers have been sleeping with their babies to keep them warm and safe from predators since the time families ate mastodons for dinner. Even if a mastodon no longer sounds as tempting as cheesecake, Dr. McKenna believes that keeping the baby close to his mother remains the natural thing to do. He explains that all babies are born physiologically "expecting" a steady stream of sensations – specifically, the touches, smells, sounds, movements, and warmth they receive only from being in close proximity to their mothers, day and night.

When these sensations cease — because one has been deposited in a separate bedroom down the hall — babies cry, signaling that something is wrong.  Dr. McKenna explains that humans are born with just 25 percent of their adult brain volume, making us the least neurologically mature of any primate species at birth.  In this sense, we are all born prematurely.  The proximity of the parent may help the infant's immature nervous system learn to self-regulate during sleep.

There is a fear that bed-sharing may result in suffocation and entrapment of babies.  The scare over this likely originated from an article published in 1996 in the journal **Lancet** that reviewed the trend of sudden deaths in infants under two months of age.[9]  The study was a *retrospective* (looking back in time) review and analysis of data collected by the U.S. Consumer Product Safety Commission (CPSC) on deaths of children less than two months of age, who were placed to sleep on adult beds.  Of the 515 infant deaths that occurred over a seven-year span, 121 (23%, or approximately 17 per year) were a result of overlaying, and 394 (77%) were due to a child getting trapped in between a bed and wall or rail.  This is really scary.  How is anybody supposed to get any sleep with such nightmarish images?  However, a recent study in Ireland (among others) suggests that sharing a place of sleep per se may not increase the risk of death, but other factors do — habitual smoking and alcohol consumption may be responsible.[10]  Yet another study warns against sleeping together with infants on sofas as a potential danger, because they can slip down into the crevice or get wedged against the back of a couch.[11]

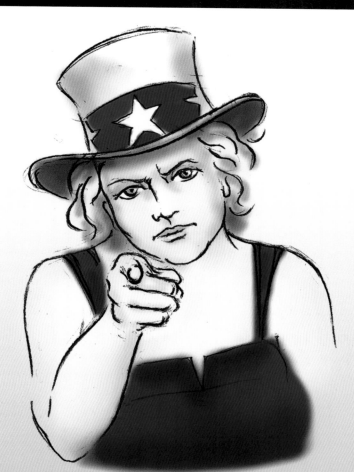

So you should not put your baby into bed
with you if you are DRUNK.

And you really should not SMOKE.

And while you may consider putting
them into the bed next to you,
you should NEVER consider putting them
into a SOFA-BED.

At this point in time, not enough is known about sudden infant death syndrome (SIDS) to make a definitive statement regarding bed-sharing in cases when there is no obvious suffocation or entrapment. Rare metabolic disorders, heart arrhythmias, and neurological problems may be responsible for many cases of SIDS.

Bed-sharing cannot be universally dangerous, because it has been practiced for centuries, and we survived. One developmental pediatrician confided that she had put all three of her babies to bed with her, because that was the only way that anybody in her family got any sleep. The practice allowed her to function as a working mother. She kept it a secret from all her colleagues, until the children were already in high school. When she revealed her secret, it turned out that several of her peers did the same thing. As for co-sleeping in the same room, unlike bed-sharing, substantial evidence exists that it is protective against SIDS. A popular new approach

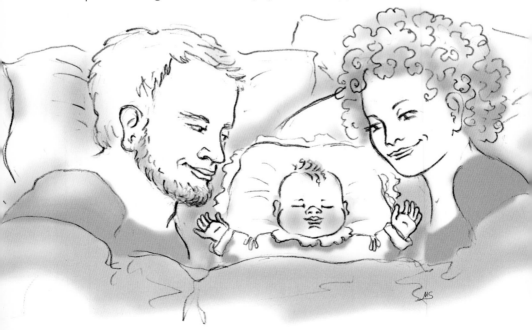

that provides all the benefits of closeness without the risks of bed-sharing is a co-sleeper: a crib that opens at the mother's bedside. It is especially trendy in Europe. Unfortunately, some anecdotal evidence suggests that some people end up using them as changing tables and then putting the baby into their bed with them anyway!

The main point is that most breastfeeding mothers find it easier to feed the baby at night, when they are in close proximity, whether in the same room or even in the same bed. You can issue all sorts of warnings; you can argue about it; but when it is two o'clock in the morning, sometimes the most primitive instincts win. Maybe this is the way that nature intended. Interestingly, mothers who co-sleep have been cited as breastfeeding twice as long as mothers who don't.

# And Now a Word on the Myth of Sleeping Through the Night

"Is your baby sleeping through the night yet?" every other parent asks anxiously. It is the most common baby question (after "Is it a boy or girl?" — even if she is dressed from head to toe in pink fluff). And when you say no, she is not sleeping through the night yet, there is only one word to describe the reaction of the other parents: SHAUDENFREUDE (German for taking delight in the misfortunes of others). Every baby is different, but it is a myth that any baby always sleeps through the night (defined as six hours). Babies teethe, get colds, and go through phases. It is not realistic to expect babies to sleep the same way every night. They are too little.

Since the majority of babies sleep through the night more often than not between the age of six months to one year, or at least wake far less frequently as they grow (and quickly go back to sleep after breastfeeding), *waiting it out* doesn't imply waiting for an eternity.

*In jumping and tumbling*
*We spend the whole day,*
*Till night by arriving*
*Has finished our play.*
*What then? One and all,*
*There's no more to be said,*
*As we tumbled all day,*
*So we tumble to bed.*

Anonymous (circa 1745), *Tumbling*

# The Secret Caveman Sleep Method: One More Alternative

Sleep experts agree on the importance of a bedtime ritual: a bath, a massage, and a story. It is a great idea. Unfortunately, by the time the baby-spa experience draws to a close, you are more tired, but the baby appears happily awake. We propose a slightly more practical variation on this theme. Our idea is to go back to cavemen times when day was day and night was night: the sunrise signaled people to wake, and the sunset signaled people to sleep. During the day, turn all lights on; make noise; clap and sing; play music. At bedtime, turn the lights off; make the house quiet; go to a room associated with sleep; cuddle with your baby and make him (her) feel snuggly and warm. Maybe nurse a while. The baby just might fall asleep, after all (and stay asleep a little longer).

# All Roads Lead to Sleep

No matter what approach you take, eventually your baby will sleep more hours, and finally, sleep through the night. And then, the time will come when your baby will be away from you a lot (this time is called adolescence). So hang in there, breastfeeding mothers! Those moments when your baby is little are precious. As Goethe's Faust exclaimed:

"To that moment I beg and pray:
You're magnificent – thus, you must stay!"

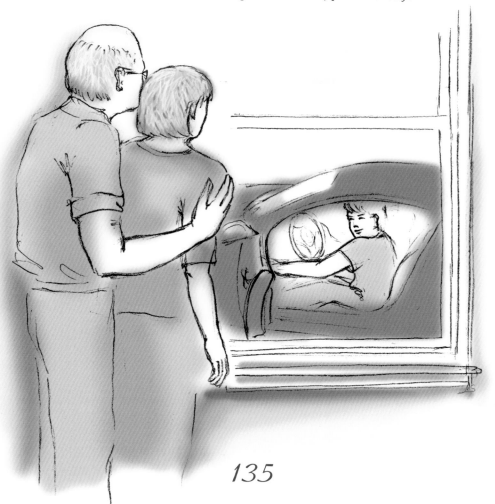

The first year is exhausting yet exhilarating. When your baby starts playing peek-a-boo; laughing when you do; clapping when you enter a room; shaking his little bottom to music; waving his finger back and forth and mischievously saying, "No, no, no!"; singing "EE-I-EE-I-O!"; making roaring sounds when asked what a lion says; and then suddenly reaching for you and giving you a kiss — LIFE IS A DREAM.

## BED-SHARING PRECAUTIONS*

Don't smoke, drink, or have too much fun first.

Don't bed-share if you or your partner sleep deeply or suffer from a sleep disorder such as apnea (deep sleepers are at risk for rolling over on the baby).

Don't EVER bed-share with babies and pets together (your bedroom should not turn into a real zoo).

Make sure that the mattress is firm (no water beds) and never share a sofa or sofa-bed for sleep.

Don't leave stuffed animals or big fluffy pillows around.

Keep the bedding light (Down with Down comforters!).

Put the baby on his back, not on his stomach, to sleep. Putting babies on their backs to sleep has successfully decreased the rate of sudden infant death by forty percent. As an aside, you may want to slightly vary the position of the baby's head from side to side, which minimizes pressure forces that cause plagiocephaly (*oblique head* in Latin). Look at the back of the head of two-month-old baby, and you will probably notice a slight flattening on one side. But rest assured, in most cases it will improve with time.

Babies can squirm and roll — never leave them on a bed unattended, or you will be sorry when you have to explain that one to the pediatrician (and even more sorry if the baby gets hurt).

Even if you follow all of these guidelines, it may still be advisable to resist your temptation to bed-share with the baby, especially for the first few months. Consider a co-sleeper: it is a safer alternative and still allows you closeness with your baby.

*Please note that AAP has issued strong statements against any bed-sharing; however, co-sleeping with the baby in the same room in a safe crib is actually favored.

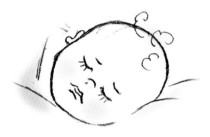

$P$ut me to bed in a hurry
For I can hardly wait
Until tomorrow morning comes
For fear I should be late.

It's so long till the morning
But if I go to bed,
I'll skip tonight, and find it is
Tomorrow, then, instead.

I've eaten all my supper
And not made any crumbs,
So now, the sooner I'm asleep
The quicker tomorrow comes.

Anna Bird Stewart, *The Night Before*

# PUMP IT UP

*(without losing your sanity)!*

$\mathcal{I}$t is ironic that while the American Academy of Pediatrics (AAP), Center for Disease Prevention and Control (CDC), and several other official sounding organizations recommend at least six months of exclusive breastfeeding (and optimally at least a year or even two of continuing breastfeeding), the majority of women in the country only get six weeks maternity leave. The short period barely provides enough time for women to recover physically let alone adjust emotionally. The irony is redoubled by the fact that the leave is often labeled officially as "disability." You have a three-day-old baby (probably, the greatest accomplishment of your life!) and you have to fill out paperwork as if you broke your leg!

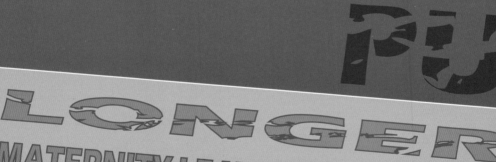

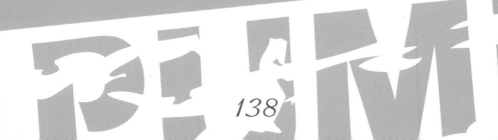

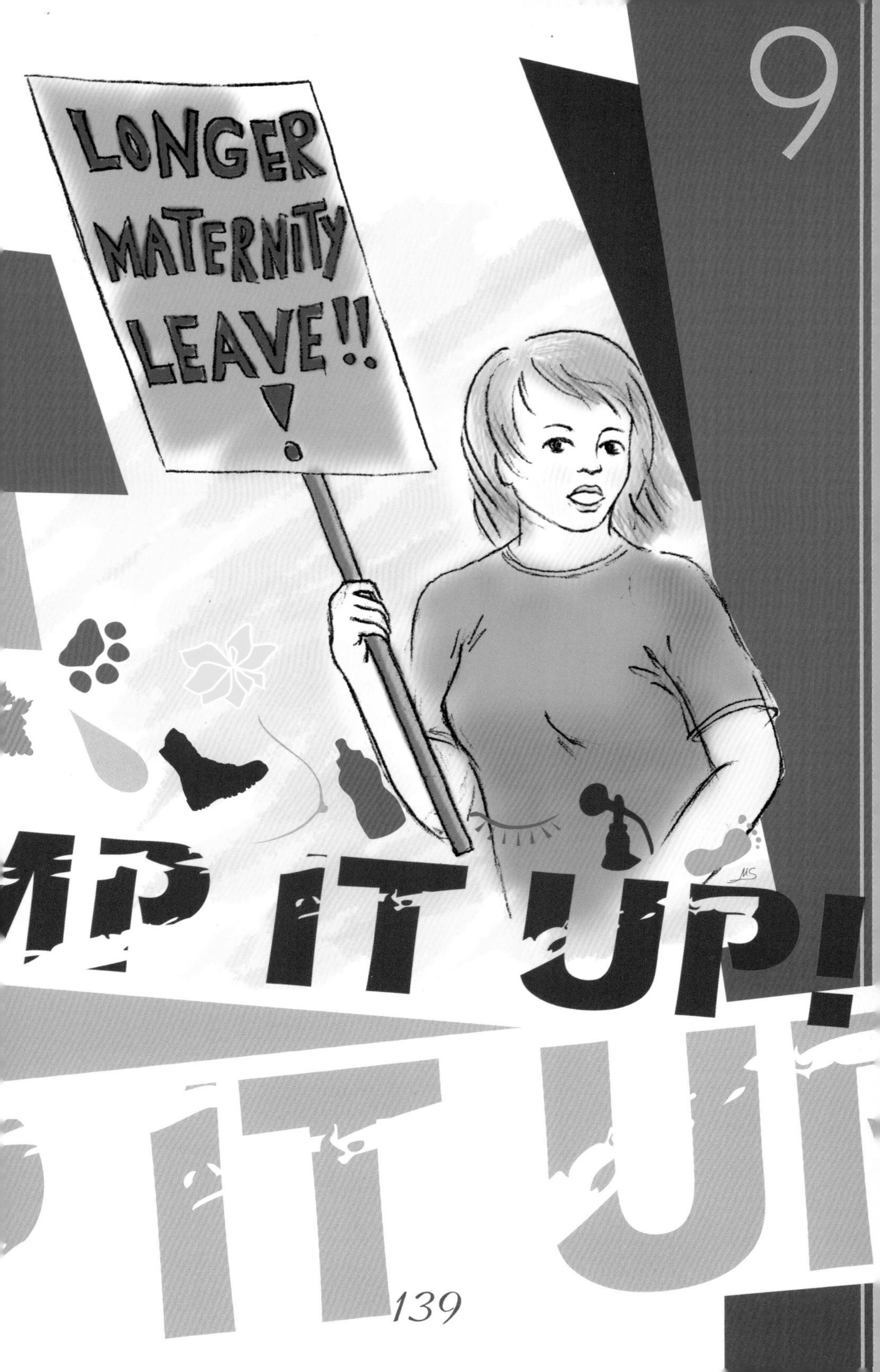

*The AAP and CDC would do far more for breastfeeding by recommending longer maternity leave first and foremost!*

Of course, the AAP, CDC, or any other three letter acronyms are not to be blamed — many of their members have lobbied Washington DC for a change in national policy. Since lawmakers are either fathers, mothers, or at least products of mothers, one would think they would be supportive of a new maternity-leave initiative. Yet they fail to pass family-oriented laws that are standard in many other parts of the world. For example, in Scandinavian countries, maternity leave is around one year. In Norway, during the twelfth month, the father gets paternity leave, while the mother returns to work. The custom is for the father to bring the baby to the mother's workplace, for she is provided with legislated breaks to breastfeed. In Russia, women get 70 days of paid leave before delivery and 70 days of paid leave after the child is born, with full wages and benefits. A mother can stay home with her baby for up to three years and receive 40% of her wages; her position is held for her during this time.

Many European countries give new mothers at least fourteen weeks of paid leave. While U.S. law mandates twelve weeks of unpaid leave, in reality, many women return to work much sooner: they can't afford to stay home, or some small companies can't afford to do without them. Naturally, many more women breastfeed in the countries like Norway or Russia than in the United States.

**Thus, it doesn't take a guideline to promote breastfeeding — it takes a real maternity leave. We need a new motto in America:**

## "Ask not what the mother can do for you, but what you can do for the mother!"

Grey-haired males, distinguished patricians,
Family values promote politicians:
Chastity, marriage, abstention, adoptions,
Teaching us, women, about these options.

Bosses demanding, colleagues condescending,
My baby is hungry and not understanding.
Milk leaks and drips through my blouse and sweater.
Life is not sweet in political theater.

Maternity leave? It's for chilly Norwegians.
In the US, we have other religions.
Lead in the toys and lobbyists' lunches,
Old boy's networks and political hunches.

Corporate filth — politicians' welfare.
Mothers, support universal childcare!
Senators, congressmen, time to take action!
Mothers, demand equal rights and protection!

M. S., *Maternity Leave*

From a mother's point of view, the prospect of leaving a six-weeks old baby at home with a nanny or in daycare is unbearable. Your baby badly needs you — after all, he is just a baby! Sometimes, he still wants to breastfeed every hour or two. Other times, he gets upset when you jump into the shower. And now you have to leave him for the entire day!?

*141*

For most of maternity leave, you barely managed to comb your hair. Now you have to take care of childcare, put on a suit and high heels, deal with paper piles on your desk, struggle against falling asleep during meetings, and try to sound articulate when nothing but the words of "itsy bitsy spider" fill your head.

> *The following joke describes the predicament of many women returning to their workplaces. "You are on an airplane, and you have made it half-way across the ocean. Suddenly, the stewardess announces: 'Ladies and Gentlemen, we are experiencing a small technical difficulty. Those of you who can swim, please proceed to the emergency exits. Those who can't, please stay in your seats. Thank you all for flying our airline, US-Jets!' "*

Fortunately, the situation is not as dire as it first seems. Mothers, you and your babies will survive! Despite the difficult adjustment period, continuing to breastfeed might be worth the extra effort. While there is nothing harder than leaving your baby in the mornings, there is nothing more gratifying than returning to your baby and immediately breastfeeding. It is a relief. Both of you will experience warmth, comfort, and reassurance of the unbreakable bond between you. In the first few weeks, the baby will want to nurse more than ever in the evenings. Eventually, however, both of you will adjust to a new routine, nursing on a more regular schedule.

In order to continue breastfeeding for a significant period of time, you have to pump at work. While other people get to *pump it up* in the gym, using savvy machines, watching TV, and listening to the rhythmic music, breastfeeding mothers *pump it up* in quite a different way. It is not exactly as becoming as a Jane Fonda work-out. The slurping machine noises, the suction cups adjusted to the woman's breasts, and the milk shooting out into collecting bottles conjure a dairy factory, not a gym. There is no getting around the fact that the first few days you will feel like a cow. However, as pumping becomes more routine, the "factory" will turn back into a cozy living room where you — a beautiful though tired woman — prepare nutritious and satisfying meals for your baby. Maybe these meals will have the flavor of the scrambled eggs that you ate for breakfast, or Chicken Parmesan you had for lunch. Pumped milk is a generous and noble gift that only a mother could offer to her baby.

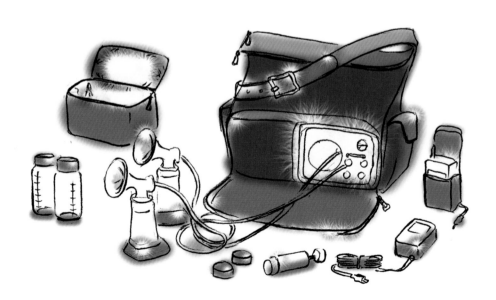

At first, pumping takes time, practice, and frequent sessions. Eventually, once or twice a day (twenty minutes in an eight-hour day) should provide enough milk. Commercials advertise that you could save a child for the price of a cup of coffee a day. In your case, for the price of a coffee break (or two), you could provide your baby with priceless food.

> My little pink rabbit fell on the floor,
> He hurt his four paws and tail,
> He sighs, he complains, he pretends he's so frail —
> But the truth is — he wants me to play with him more.

Agnia Barto, *My Little Pink Rabbit*

Luckily, your labor is significantly reduced with the help of an electric breast pump, which not only allows both breasts to empty simultaneously but also comes in a stylish backpack that you port around the office. People who do not realize its hidden function will invariably give you compliments: "Great new bag!" Mothers who breastfed will recognize it and give reassuring glances or thumbs-up signs.

The pump contains a removable cooler unit, collection containers and lids, suction cups (the parts that go on the breast), an electric outlet adaptor, a battery pack, and tubing. A good strategy is to buy extra bottles and suction cups, because those are the parts that have to be cleaned regularly.

144

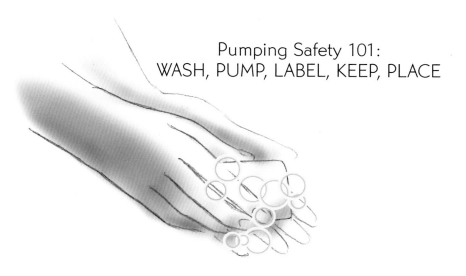

# Pumping Safety 101:
## WASH, PUMP, LABEL, KEEP, PLACE

WASH hands before pumping.

If you plan to freeze the milk, PUMP into special plastic bags which are attached straight to suction cups (available at any baby store or on-line).

If you plan to refrigerate the milk or offer it to your baby soon, PUMP straight into bottles.

If your child goes to a day-care, LABEL the bag or bottle with today's date and your child's name (lest she gets somebody else's breast milk).

KEEP fresh and frozen milk separate.

PLACE frozen milk into the refrigerator to thaw it in advance. If you need to use it quickly, PLACE it into a bowl of warm water. Avoid refreezing thawed milk.

MOST IMPORTANTLY: never use a microwave to thaw frozen milk, since you can burn the baby with a pocket of scalding milk!

# The Pumping Diaries: A Week in the Life

This is the life of a breastfeeding, working, pumping mother:

In the morning, she feeds her baby just before leaving. The night before, she has sterilized four bottles (placed in the cooler carrier) and four suction cups (placed in the storage compartment of the bag). Now, she remembers to add the freezer pack to the removable cooler carrier; if she is lucky, she grabs something to eat, and runs out of the house.

During her busy day, she tries to pump two times, once for fifteen minutes at lunch-time, and once during an afternoon coffee-break. Both times, she stores the milk in the freezer pack. When she arrives home, the baby smiles and kicks when he sees her but cries if she doesn't immediately pick him up. She throws the milk into the refrigerator, the ice pack into the freezer, washes her hands, and then joyously hugs her baby.

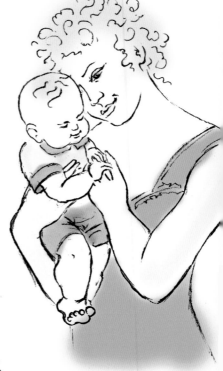

The baby breastfeeds and looks delighted; the mother and baby enjoy the best moment of the day. After the mother breastfeeds him a few more times, plays with him, and changes his diapers (hopefully with some help from dad or well-meaning relatives), the baby falls asleep.

This is often the mother's only time to catch-up on phone calls, bills, e-mails, and to try to get herself and household together. Sometimes, she manages to eat something, maybe leftovers or a spoonful of ice cream. Then, she collapses into bed.

A few more times during the night she wakes to feed her baby, and in no time (time flies when we are having fun!) she is ready for work. That schedule remains the same at least five days a week. Legislators who ignore bills for longer maternity leaves should try a breastfeeding mother's schedule out, even though it might interfere with dinner with the lobbyists.

Five days a week, a typical breastfeeding mother encounters and overcomes the following obstacles:

**Obstacle One: An absence of room (and privacy) to pump.** Some inventive mothers will go as far as pumping in a locker room, ladies room, or their parked car (but never while driving, because the mother's safety matters more to the baby than anything else in the world, including breast milk). Recently, a female friend, who is an obstetrician, mentioned that several of her colleagues have even begun pumping during meetings — *a step beyond breastfeeding in public!* This might be the start of a revolution in the corporate world! However, you definitely should stop short of pouring your milk into the boss' coffee!!

**Obstacle Two: A lack of support from colleagues.** Unfortunately, not all women work with fellow pediatricians, who promote breastfeeding and uniformly offer support. Many women experience sneers or hostile attitudes from their supervisors or colleagues (especially if they need the private use of a shared office), who think that pumping causes interference with the professional day. Ironically, these colleagues are likely to spend far more time on browsing the web or talking rash.

Many breastfeeding mothers manage to pump, send e-mails, or return phone calls, all at the same time. Some even use a special hands-free tube bra (available via the internet) that clasps the pumps in place (undoubtedly some breastfeeding mother's invention). With a little practice, a less-expensive maternity bra can also snap around the suction cups and hold them to leave hands free for phone calls or typing. Breastfeeding mothers are the ultimate multi-taskers.

Mothers who breastfeed have on average fewer sick days than mothers who do not, since their babies usually get ill less often. Thus, more savvy workplaces have begun encouraging pumping by providing pumping rooms with comfortable chairs and magazines. Maybe some day, these rooms will replace bars as the top spots for making business deals!

**Obstacle Three: Breast engorgement and leaking milk in the first few weeks returning to work.** You talk to your supervisor or other colleagues, when you suddenly notice strange looks. You look down

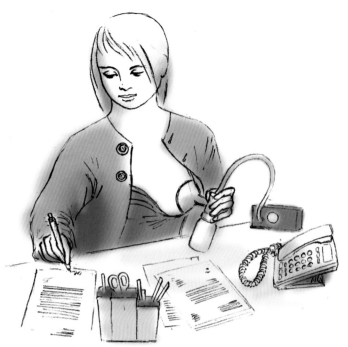

and see that your shirt is getting wet. The embarrassment is indescribable. Breast pads, a change of clothes, and in particular, a sense of humor help. It is also useful to avoid looking at cute baby pictures (especially yours), which send milk pouring out! Remember, there is a connection between the heart, the brain, and the breast!

**Obstacle Four: A drastic decrease in milk supply, especially in times of stress.** The mother feels as though the milk has gone forever. Later, when trying to wean, women find that — for better or worse — breast milk doesn't just poof away. During times when supply is low, drinking a lot of water and eating more food to increase caloric intake help. People recommend various milk-boosting cocktails, from raspberry tea to premium Irish beer. Some swear by almond butter and ice cream. Anything delicious is worth trying. What invariably succeeds is increasing frequency of pumping (it is not necessary to increase the time per session); in most cases, after a few days, a normal milk supply returns. In the interim, freezer stores of pumped milk or formula can obviously be used. If only there was a solution that permanently reduced stress!

**Obstacle Five: Pumped milk left on the counter.** The first thing that you see when you come home is a bottle of your pumped milk spoiling on the counter, inevitably forgotten by your babysitter or husband. If other people appreciated how you labored over every ounce of milk, they would treat this milk like Russians treat their beluga caviar. But we can't blame them too much, since these people have spent the day heating up the milk, carrying bulky strollers, changing diapers, singing to try to get your baby to sleep, and praying for your safe and speedy return. And when you finally make it home, just remember, "Don't cry over spilled milk!" (even your own).

## *Heroic efforts*

*Some breastfeeding mothers* say that they pumped for a month or so after returning to work, and then they couldn't stand it anymore. They still continued nursing in the morning and evening and supplemented with formula the rest of the time. *Other mothers* breastfed exclusively until the first birthday, and then they threw the pump victoriously into the sea (or only the tubing into the sea and the pump deep into a dark closet for the next baby). *Still other breastfeeding mothers*, after trials and tribulations and hard working conditions, quit breastfeeding. Any of these efforts are heroic. Who else would do what a mother does for her baby?!

# IDEAS THAT MAKE PUMPING EASIER
## (OR AT LEAST MAKE YOU FEEL BETTER)

1. Breastfeed your baby right before you leave for work and immediately when you come home. This keeps your milk supply up.

2. Remember to drink a lot of water and eat well.

3. Use breast pads and store a change of clothes at work or a big coat for cover-ups, in case you leak.

4. Aside from the pump, buy an extra set of tubing and suction cups; then bring each set in a separate plastic bag – you can simply use a fresh set for each session.

5. A microwave can save a lot of time when you sterilize baby's bottles, but never use a microwave to heat frozen milk.

6. To increase milk supply, try Raspberry tea, beer (one glass is probably alright when breastfeeding), almond butter (consider avoiding nuts if you have a family history of food allergies), and ice cream. There is no medical evidence that these alternatives work, but they are certainly delicious!

7. Store some extra milk in the freezer: if your supply goes down, use the stores while increasing the frequency of pumping over the next few days. Consider pumping once a day during the last few weeks of your maternity leave.

8. Aim to pump in a 24 hour period about as much milk as the baby takes when you are away.

9. If you pump in the evening, during the night, or on weekends, one concern is that this will deplete your breasts of milk exactly when your baby wants to eat. In actuality, this rarely happens, because the baby is better at extracting milk than even the best pump.

10. In later months, consider leaving the pump at work (and just taking home the tubing, suction cups, freezer pack, and pumped milk), so you don't have to lug it back and forth. Another alternative is to leave the electric pump at work and use a cheaper manual pump at home if extra sessions are needed.

*151*

# STORAGE DURATION OF FRESH HUMAN MILK FOR USE WITH HEALTHY FULL TERM INFANTS[12]

| Location | Temperature | Duration | Comments |
|---|---|---|---|
| Countertop, table | Room temperature (up to 77°F or 25°C) | 6-8 hours | Containers should be covered and kept as cool as possible; covering the container with a cool towel may keep milk cooler. |
| Insulated cooler bag | 5-39°F or -15-4°C | 24 hours | Keep ice packs in contact with milk containers at all times, limit opening cooler bag. |
| Refrigerator | 39°F or 4°C | 5 days | Store milk in the back of the main body of the refrigerator. |
| Freezer compartment of refrigerator with separate doors | 0°F or -18°C | 3-6 months | Store milk toward the back of the freezer, where temperature is most constant. Milk stored for longer durations in the ranges listed is safe, but some of the lipids in the milk undergo degradation resulting in lower quality. |

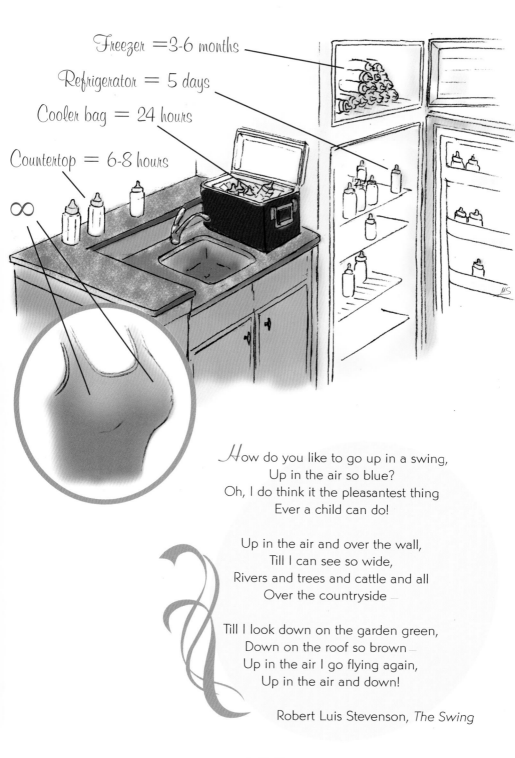

Freezer = 3-6 months

Refrigerator = 5 days

Cooler bag = 24 hours

Countertop = 6-8 hours

∞

How do you like to go up in a swing,
Up in the air so blue?
Oh, I do think it the pleasantest thing
Ever a child can do!

Up in the air and over the wall,
Till I can see so wide,
Rivers and trees and cattle and all
Over the countryside —

Till I look down on the garden green,
Down on the roof so brown —
Up in the air I go flying again,
Up in the air and down!

Robert Luis Stevenson, *The Swing*

# WEAN LIKE A WINNER

## *(and toast to making it through)!*

*M*other seals have it easy. They suckle their pups for only four days. Even though they live at sea, they must give birth and nurse out of the water. The only

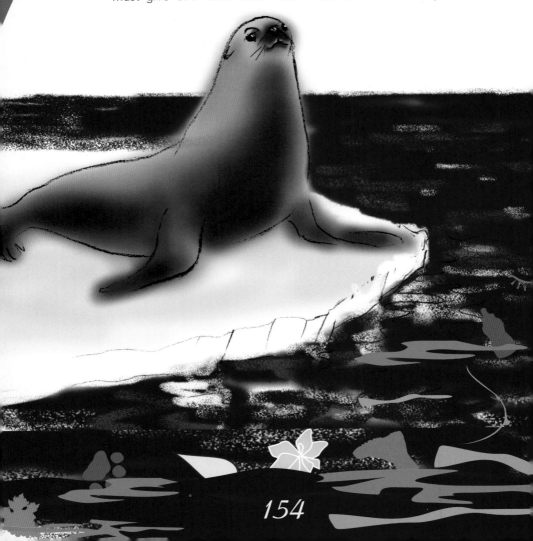

surface available is floating ice.  A storm could
break the ice into pieces and crush the mother;
or an ice floe might split, separating a mother
from her pups.  Thus, the short nursing period
(the shortest of any mammal) helps baby seals
survive.  The milk that they get is so high in fat
that they gain enough strength and insulation to
live in a polar environment after only four days
of breastfeeding.

Modern women live in a different climate.
It is unclear exactly how long our babies need

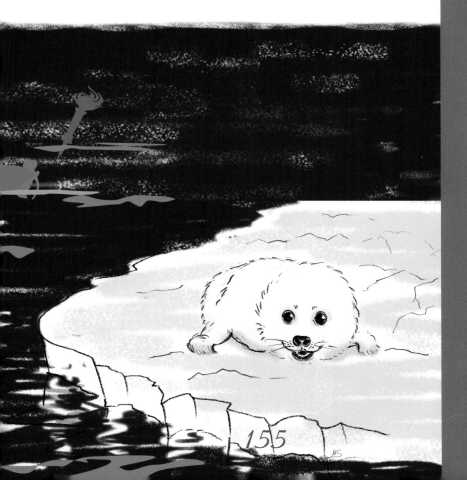

155

breast milk or when to wean them. Every woman is on her own.

Clearly, the majority of women in America stop breastfeeding at some point in the first year. Those of us who make it to six months or breastfeed exclusively for a year have done something exceptional. But we too cannot go on forever. Maybe it is too hard to pump at work. Maybe we want our breasts back to ourselves, so that we can wear a nice dress without buttons that rip open at a moment's notice, enjoy a double espresso, or sip a strawberry daiquiri on a lounge chair on the beach. Mothers are people too.

Of course, we'll miss nursing: when our baby falls, wakes at night, or teethes, breastfeeding soothes her.

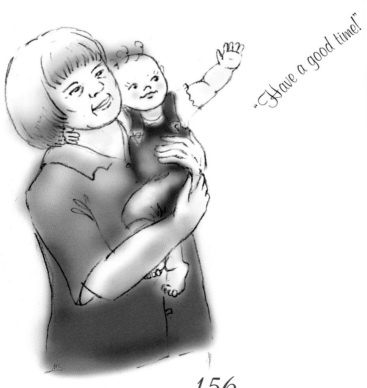

"Have a good time!"

She looks so joyous afterwards, making clicking noises or clapping. It is hard to imagine taking that source of happiness and comfort away. Plus, when we separate from our babies and pumps, our breasts get engorged. How is a mother to stop, when her baby and even her body want to hold on?

Some mothers don't. They sing the mantra "You can breastfeed as long as you want to!" It is a testament to how much babies love breastfeeding that many don't wean on their own little accords. In many countries,

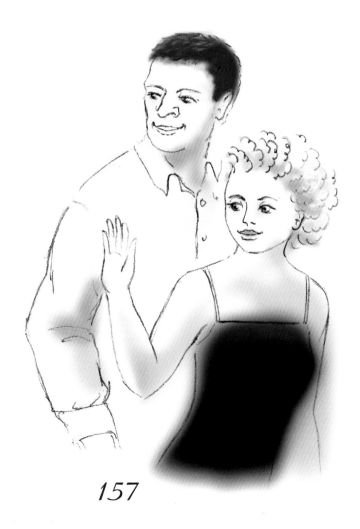

it is normal to breastfeed a toddler. In America where "anything goes," from piercing in discreet parts of the body to body art, surely breastfeeding a few months longer than average should not raise too many brows. This is called "child-led, or natural weaning." There are health and other benefits to continuing, but when the child reaches a certain age, even the most patient mothers may want to stop: "Now Nadia, if you don't nurse, I will give you a chocolate chip cookie, or how about a nice doll?" Rest assured, baby-led weaning (or bribery) works eventually, since nobody breastfeeds in college.

Still other mothers say enough is enough and prefer stopping abruptly. Maybe they blow out the first-year birthday candles and say that is it. Or, they go back to a high-intensity job where they cannot pump. For several days, these women may endure engorgement, chills, and sometimes even fever due to rapidly changing hormones. The risk to the mother is that abrupt weaning may lead to her experiencing PMS-type symptoms magnified, if not clinical depression. A few days of raw cabbage leaves, cold compresses, and tears pass, and then life goes on. Nurse from *Romeo and Juliet* weaned Juliet abruptly (Juliet was almost three-years old though). From Shakespeare's point of view, it was painless and comical, of course!

_And she was weaned – I never shall forget it –
Of all the days of the year upon that day.
For I had then laid wormwood to my dug, [breast]
Sitting in the sun under the dovehouse wall. . .
When it [Juliet] did taste the wormwood on the nipple
Of my dug and felt it bitter, pretty fool,
To see it tetchy and fall out with the dug.

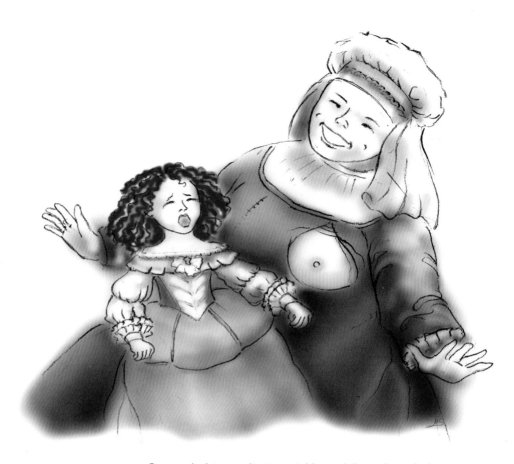

Some babies adjust quickly, while other babies refuse formula or whole milk in protest. The *"cry it out"* approach is best reserved for cases of personal or medical necessity.

Somewhere in between baby-led weaning and abrupt weaning is gradual weaning. Women set a breastfeeding goal of either six months or a year. At a certain point, they gradually replace one feeding a week with formula (before one year), whole-milk (after a year), and perhaps some solids (after six months). The morning and evening feeds are the last to go. Both mother and baby make it through without major trauma.

# A Time to Wean

In biblical times, weaning was celebrated. In our busy and hectic life, the breastfeeding era often ends anti-climatically: we have lost the sense of weaning as a process of spiritual renewal for the mother, as well as growth and independence for the baby.

The definition of weaning is the introduction of food other than breast milk, and the normally recommended time to start that introduction is around six months. Six months is a magical time for a baby in a sense: many babies are sitting up on their own, lose their tongue thrust (which makes them gag when taking food), and seem especially curious about putting everything in their mouths. As an aside, this is also a nice time for the mother, since a six-month-old baby is easier to take on longer excursions; he is more interested in the world; and he is often a little more independent. It is the perfect time to leave him with dad or a relative for an hour and take a bike ride or try an alternatively popular exercise: shopping!

Remember, according to the American Academy of Pediatrics (AAP), World Health Organization (WHO), Center for Disease Prevention and Control (CDC), and every official sounding agency (OSA), babies should be breastfed exclusively for the first half-year. And when they say "exclusively," they mean it in a hard-line way. Not one sip of water (even in the sweltering heat). The argument is that breast milk is over eighty percent water anyway, and babies need the extra nutrients for optimal growth and development. Also, delaying solids decreases the risk of allergies.

Sometimes guidelines are hard to follow. Of course, it is not a good idea to use water (or chamomile tea, and all the other things that relatives offer) as a supplement, especially in the first few months. However, giving a tiny bit of water to a four-month-old to get her used to the idea of a sippy cup seems acceptable.

## First Food (Mush) Fun Time

Many people make a big fuss about what food to introduce first. The exact choice varies in most countries in the world. It is really a matter of consistency rather than substance. Almost any mush made just a bit thicker than liquid works. Rice cereal is easy; fresh banana mixed with breast milk or water is another favorite. Ripe avocado

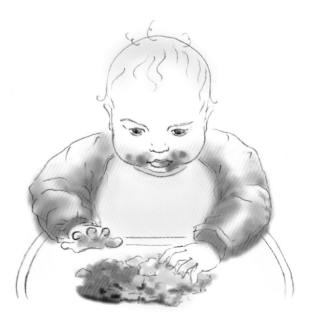

blended with water is delicious and healthy. Stage I baby carrots are convenient. It is a great joy to spoon-feed your baby and watch him spread orange gook all over his face. The traditional paradigm of always doing cereal, vegetables, fruit, and meat in a religious order still works, but there is nothing wrong with changing the order (in fact, that is the latest trend). Some families eventually get to the point of throwing every meal that they eat (even pizza) into the blender for the baby and calling it a day!

Before the baby is set for pizza, he might turn away or reject the spoon, which means he is not ready. In most cases, months six through nine are spent with babies eating complete mush, often in a disinterested way. And then something interesting happens. Your baby gets teeth, lifts off the floor in a bear-crawl, stands with support, and starts looking truly like a little person. One night, you are eating zucchini and spaghetti with the baby sitting on your lap, and suddenly she grabs it and chews a whole piece!

Now, it is time to have fun and to start introducing a variety of foods, maybe even offering a little three times a day. People talk about waiting a week in between every new food (in case an allergic reaction takes place), but there is little direct evidence that it makes a great difference. The idea is not to introduce a million things at once, but if you happen to give squash and potatoes together, there is usually no harm. And you don't have to mark the calendar with days and times to introduce new foods: you could have some flexibility. Of course, if there is a family history of food allergies or a previous reaction, a more cautious approach is needed. The most common reaction is a skin rash, and an extra big diaper rash may also be a sign. In this case, you should consult the pediatrician yet again!

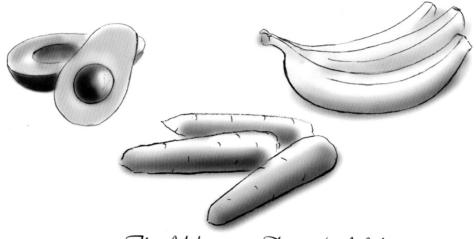

# The Weaning Diet (A Variant of the Breastfeeding Diet)

During pregnancy and breastfeeding, most of us splurged on strawberry milkshakes and plates of Fettuccini Alfredo. Now your baby is ready to eat solids. Does that mean you have to cook something special for her? Not if you follow "the weaning diet," which allows you to eliminate the need to cook different meals for different members of the family. The main idea is that you, your baby, and entire family can enjoy a lot of the same foods. As your baby gets more interested in solids, especially between 10-12 months, you gradually cut down on the amount of breast milk consumed by the baby during the day, and substitute breast milk with the food you too like to eat. Weaning is cooking.

# TOP FIVE BREAKFAST OPTIONS THAT YOU AND YOUR BABY CAN SHARE

**Caveat:** get the green light from your pediatrician or proceed at your own risk!

1) Oatmeal and pears. Peel and cut a pear in small pieces; add the pear to a small saucepan filled with half-water and half-organic apple juice; when it comes to a boil, add about four large handfuls of oats; cook fifteen minutes or so until the whole thing is mushy (YUM!).

2) Eggs (your baby ONLY gets the yolk). Separate one egg, scramble the yolk in a little butter or olive oil on the pan first and cut it into tiny pieces for the baby. Mix the remaining egg white with some more eggs and scramble for the rest of the family.

3) Whole yogurt and bananas. Mash with a fork or make a Smoothie.

4) Cheerios with breast milk for the baby (and regular milk for you).

5) Organic applesauce with whole-grain bread (made into crumbs for your baby, toasted for you).

The friendly cow, all red and white,
I love with all my heart:
She gives me cream with all her might,
To eat with apple-tart.

She wanders lowing here and there,
And yet she cannot stray.
All in the pleasant open air,
The pleasant light of day;

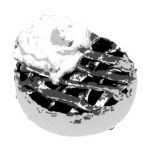

And blown by all the winds that pass
And wet with all the showers,
She walks among the meadow grass
And eat the meadow flowers.

Robert Louis Stevenson, *The Cow*

## TOP FIVE LUNCH OPTIONS

1) Avocado sandwiches. Mash the avocado and crumb the bread for your baby; for you, mix with low-fat cottage cheese, lemon juice, and salt and pepper for a delicious spread.

2) Hummus. Take a can of chick peas, puree in the blender with a tablespoon or so of olive oil; take out a few tablespoons for the baby; then for you, add ¼ cup of lemon juice, 1/3 cup of tahini or sesame seeds, salt and pepper; and add cilantro, parsley, or any other herb, if you have it on hand. Put on pita for you and it's fabulous!

3) Baked potatoes or sweet potatoes. Stab with a fork, microwave for five minutes, turn over, microwave for five minutes more: for the baby peel the skin, and mash it up!

4) Fruit-salad. Choose from extra-ripe papaya, persimmon, honeydew, cantaloupe, and bananas. It should be ripe enough to easily mash with a fork. Eat yours with cottage cheese, yogurt, or as is.

5) Yummy Cauliflower. Steam for fifteen minutes for you, for a few minutes longer for your baby. Mash a few soft heads with a potatoes masher for the baby or throw in a blender. For you, add bread crumbs, a little butter or melted cheese, and you are all set! And make yourself a salad.

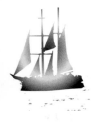

When I was down beside the sea
A wooden spade they gave to me
To dig the sandy shore.

My holes were empty like a cup,
In every hole the sea came up,
Till it could come no more.

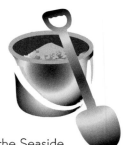

Robert Louis Stevenson, At the Seaside

## TOP FIVE DINNER OPTIONS

1) Super-mashed beans. Soak beans such as lima or red beans overnight. The next day drain the water, rinse them, add a can of tomato paste, diced tomatoes, a few tablespoons of olive oil, salt and pepper, and fill the pot half-way with water. Cook on the back-burner for several hours. When serving to your baby, make sure that the beans are all mashed up (use a potatoes masher). Serve with rice made in a rice-cooker, add a salad, and dinner is

ready for the family (and don't forget hot sauce for the table)!

2) Spaghetti and zucchini. Sauté four thinly sliced zucchinis in just a little olive oil in a large pan for ten minutes (or until the pieces are very soft and clear). Meanwhile, prepare the spaghetti according to package instructions. When it is ready, take the majority of it out, but leave your baby's portion for about three minutes longer. Take out four or five pieces of zucchini, peal their skin, and cut into small pieces; add some of the super soft spaghetti cut up into tiny pieces. For your portion, mix the al dente spaghetti with the rest of the zucchini and add some parmesan cheese.

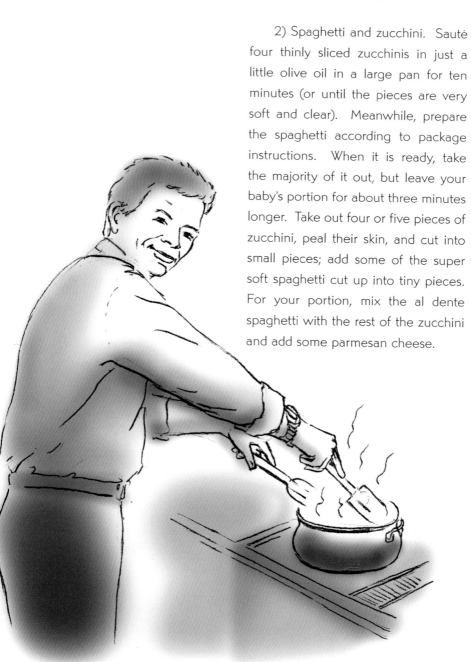

3) Tofu with mixed vegetables. Thinly slice a package of baby carrots, a zucchini, and some squash. Sauté with a little olive oil or butter, while slicing the tofu. After about fifteen minutes, throw in the tofu – once it is hot, you are set! Mash your baby's portion with a fork. If the vegetables are well-cooked, the baby can eat small pieces.

4) Broiled wild (not farm-raised) boneless salmon with broccoli. Broil salmon with a little olive oil for seven minutes on each side. Cut some flakes and triple-check for bones for your baby's portion. Wash broccoli and steam for seven minutes for you; an additional five minutes for the baby. Blend your baby's portion in the blender or use a potatoes masher on the heads.

5) Ground turkey balls with potatoes. Wash a package of ground meat; sauté an onion; mix along with one raw egg and a few handfuls of oats; add salt and pepper; form meatballs and fry in olive oil. Make potatoes any way that you know!

At dusk, when it is very still,
I think I am alone until
The little child I used to be
Comes in to sit and talk with me.

I see beyond her, through the haze,
All my forgotten yesterdays.
I'm glad we know each other yet,
I, and the child we can't forget.

Anna Bird Stewart, *Envoy*

# The Final Stages of Weaning

The first part of weaning, which involves simply introducing foods and replacing breast milk, is natural and fun. The second part of weaning, cutting out breastfeeding completely, is sometimes more challenging. While some babies easily lose interest in breastfeeding, other babies remain staunchly attached, especially to evening and morning feeds. For those avid breastfeeders, distraction helps. Silly songs, pantomimes, games of catch, car rides, and the outdoors offer diversions from the breast!!

# A Still Breastfeeding Mother's Story

I stopped pumping when my baby turned one, thinking that my baby would wean shortly after. But it so happened that she still held on to morning and evening feeds.

For the most part, I no longer nursed her during the day, but I relented on an especially hot afternoon in Brighton Beach, while visiting a friend. My baby had spent the day playing in the sand, running into the water and back, and riding on a carousel. There was too much excitement for a nap. Suddenly, she was desperately tired and thirsty. I sat down on the nearest bench and tried to cover up with my sun-hat.

"GOD - Just look at that mother nursing such a BIG girl," I heard one woman say loudly to another. It took me a second to realize that my little baby (at fifteen months) appeared like a "big girl" from an objective perspective. She was still so tiny and helpless in my eyes.

Their reaction made me wonder if this breastfeeding business had gone on for too long. Maybe it was time for another step — to start a breastfeeding anonymous in order to quit. But unlike other vices, breastfeeding seemed a relatively harmless (and even healthy one) to permit.

There were times when I tried to distract my baby from nursing with games; or by offering her spoons of creamy whole milk; slowing down the nursing sessions; and even holding out chocolate ice-cream. She would demand nursing instead but afterwards remember the ice-cream to eat. She always won.

Sometimes, in the middle of nursing, my baby would raise her head, look at me mischievously, and then quickly resume; sometimes she would laugh or sigh with great satisfaction upon finishing; and other times, she would fall asleep in the most dreamy way, with her mouth slightly open and curls around her cheeks.

Maybe she breastfed at this point more for comfort and habit than for sustenance. Maybe she breastfed because she missed me during my long working day, and breastfeeding allowed her to feel closeness again. Or maybe she just liked it. Why should I take such a simple joy away?

I don't really know how to wean as a winner. Surely, that doesn't mean that I can't toast to making it through! Breastfeeding is action, a unique marathon with a self-defined course and finish line!

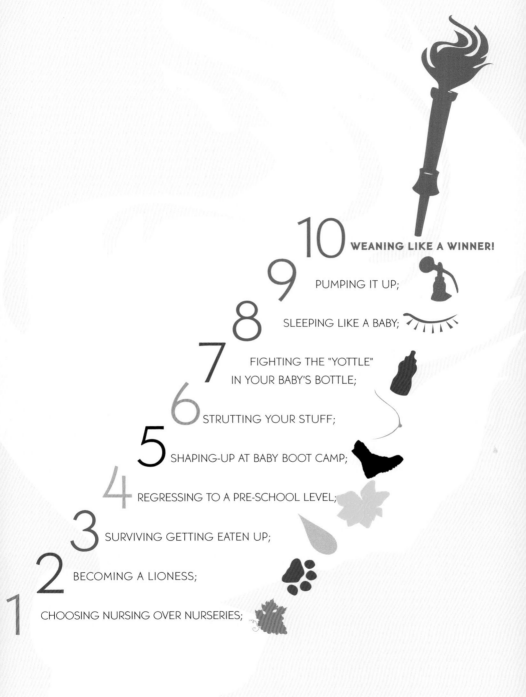

10 **WEANING LIKE A WINNER!**

9   PUMPING IT UP;

8   SLEEPING LIKE A BABY;

7   FIGHTING THE "YOTTLE"
IN YOUR BABY'S BOTTLE;

6   STRUTTING YOUR STUFF;

5   SHAPING-UP AT BABY BOOT CAMP;

4   REGRESSING TO A PRE-SCHOOL LEVEL;

3   SURVIVING GETTING EATEN UP;

2   BECOMING A LIONESS;

1   CHOOSING NURSING OVER NURSERIES;

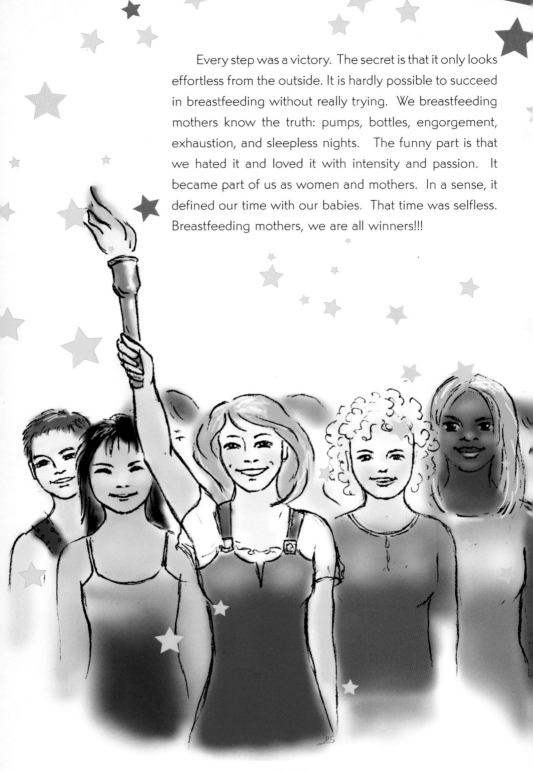

Every step was a victory. The secret is that it only looks effortless from the outside. It is hardly possible to succeed in breastfeeding without really trying. We breastfeeding mothers know the truth: pumps, bottles, engorgement, exhaustion, and sleepless nights. The funny part is that we hated it and loved it with intensity and passion. It became part of us as women and mothers. In a sense, it defined our time with our babies. That time was selfless. Breastfeeding mothers, we are all winners!!!

172

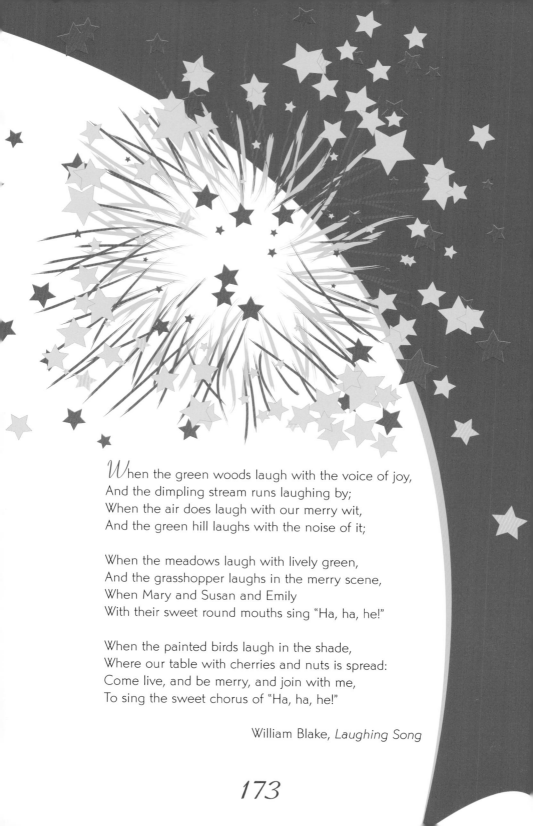

When the green woods laugh with the voice of joy,
And the dimpling stream runs laughing by;
When the air does laugh with our merry wit,
And the green hill laughs with the noise of it;

When the meadows laugh with lively green,
And the grasshopper laughs in the merry scene,
When Mary and Susan and Emily
With their sweet round mouths sing "Ha, ha, he!"

When the painted birds laugh in the shade,
Where our table with cherries and nuts is spread:
Come live, and be merry, and join with me,
To sing the sweet chorus of "Ha, ha, he!"

William Blake, *Laughing Song*

# References:

[1] http://www.cdc.gov/breastfeeding/data/infant_feeding.htm

[2] J. A. César, C. G. Victora, F. C. Barros, I. S. Santos, J. A. Flores, Impact of breast feeding on admission for pneumonia during postneonatal period in Brazil: nested case-control study, *British Medical Journal*. **318** (7194), 1316-1320 (1999).

[3] J. L. Freudenheim, J. R. Marshall, S. Graham, R. Laughlin, J. E. Vena, E. Bandera, P. Muti, M. Swanson, T. Nemoto, Exposure to breastmilk in infancy and the risk of breast cancer, *Epidemiology*. **5** (3), 324-31 (1994). Comment in: *Epidemiology*. **6** (2), 198-200 (1995).

[4] Niels H. Lauersen, M.D., Ph.D. and Eileen Stukane, *The Complete Book of Breast Care*, pp. 13-16, 29-30 (Fawcett Columbine, 1998)

[5] R. Michael Akers, Lactation and the Mammary Gland, Table – p. 78 (Wiley-Blackwell, 2002)

[6] N. E. Wight, Donor human milk for preterm infants, J Perinatol. 21 (4), 249-254 (2001).

[7] G. C. Anderson, E. Moore, J. Hepworth, N. Bergman, Early Skin-To-Skin Contact for Mothers and Their Healthy Newborn Infants, *Birth*. **30** (3), 206-207 (2) (Blackwell Publishing, 2003).

[8] J. McKenna, T. McDade, Why babies should never sleep alone: a review of the co-sleeping controversy in relation to SIDS, bedsharing and breastfeeding, *Paediatric Respiratory Reviews*. **6** (2), 134-152 (2005).

[9] E. A. Mitchell, Co-sleeping and sudden infant death syndrome, *Lancet*. **348** (9040), 1466 (1996).

[10] J. F. Glasgow, A. J. Thompson, P. J. Ingram, Sudden unexpected death in infancy: place and time of death, *Ulster Med J.* **75**(1), 65-71 (2006).

[11] P. Blair, P. Sidebotham, P. Berry, M. Evans, P. Fleming, Major epidemiological changes in sudden infant death syndrome: a 20-year-population-based study in the UK, *Lancet.* 367 (9507), 314-319 (2006).

[12] Human Milk Storage Information for Home Use for Healthy Full-Term Infants, *Academy of Breastfeeding Medicine.* (Princeton Junction, NJ (2004).

## Acknowledgement:

The authors want to express their deep gratitude for permission to use E V Rieu poem "The Paint Box." The poem was reprinted "By permission of the Authors Licensing and Collecting Society Ltd on behalf of the estate of the late E V Rieu."

**Natasha Shur**, M.D. is a diplomate of the American Board of Pediatrics and a diplomate of the American College of Medical Genetics. She received her M.D. from Albert Einstein College of Medicine in New York. She completed her residency in pediatrics and fellowship in genetics at Montefiore Medical Center in New York. She currently works as a clinical geneticist and teaches medical students at an academic hospital.

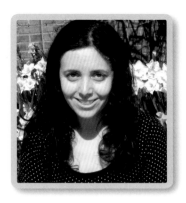

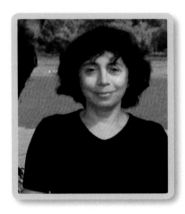

**Paulina Shur**, Theatre and Film Director, received her Ph.D. in Theatre and Film Arts from the Institute of Theatre, Music, and Film in St. Petersburg, Russia, and an M.F.A. in Theatre Directing from the University of Virginia in Charlottesville, Va. She was a founder and Artistic Director of the *Magic Mirror Theatre* in Charlottesville, Virginia, and taught theatre and film classes at Rensselaer Polytechnic Institute in Troy, NY. She currently writes, directs, and produces short films.

**Marianna Simina**, Graphic Designer and Artist, received her degree in Graphic Design from the University of South Carolina in Columbia, SC. She exhibits her works at Columbia Museum of Art, colleges, and state exhibitions. She receives awards for her portraits and is commissioned to do murals, portraits, paintings, and graphic works. Currently she works as a Graphic Designer in Columbia, SC.

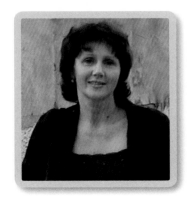